E. Martin P. Nawroth (Hrsg.)

Fachübergreifende Aspekte der Hämostaseologie IV

Springer
Berlin
Heidelberg
New York
Barcelona
Hongkong
London
Mailand
Paris
Singapur
Tokio

Eike Martin Peter Nawroth (Hrsg.)

Fachübergreifende Aspekte der Hämostaseologie IV

6. Heidelberger Symposium Hämostaseologie und Anaesthesie, 17. März 1999

Mit 20 Abbildungen und 21 Tabellen

Springer

Professor Dr. med. Eike Martin
Universität Heidelberg
Klinik für Anästhesiologie
Im Neuenheimer Feld 110
D-69120 Heidelberg

Professor Dr. med. Peter Nawroth
Universitätsklinikum Tübingen
Sektion Vaskuläre Medizin
Medizinische Klinik IV
und Poliklinik
Otfried-Müller-Straße 10
D-72076 Tübingen

ISBN 3-540-66317-7 Springer-Verlag Berlin Heidelberg New York

Die Deutsche Bibliothek – CIP-Einheitsaufnahme
Fachübergreifende Aspekte der Hämostaseologie / Eike Martin, Peter Nawroth (Hrsg.). – Berlin ; Heidelberg ; New York ; Barcelona ; Hongkong ; London ; Mailand ; Paris ; Singapur ; Tokio : Springer 4. (1999)
ISBN 3-540-66317-7

Herstellung: PRO EDIT GmbH, D-69126 Heidelberg
Umschlaggestaltung: design & production GmbH, Heidelberg
Satz: Zechner Datenservice und Druck, D-67346 Speyer

SPIN: 10737934 18/3134-5 4 3 2 1 0 – Gedruckt auf säurefreiem Papier

Vorwort

Die Sepsis ist das Ergebnis eines Krankheitsprozesses, dessen Werdegang noch kaum verstanden wird. Pathophysiologische Veränderungen, die bei der Sepsis bekannt sind, sind fast genauso, nur eben lokalisiert, z. B. auch bei einem banalen „Pickel" beschrieben.

Zytokine, Chemokine, oxidativer Streß, Aktivierung bestimmter Transkriptionsfaktoren unterscheiden sich bei „banalen" entzündlichen Krankheitsprozessen im Prinzip nicht von lebensbedrohlichen Zuständen wie der Sepsis. Es kommt zur Induktion von Genen, deren Produkte Leukozytenadhäsion vermehren, weitere Zytokine und Kaskaden der Apoptose induzieren, oxidativen Streß lokal und disseminiert vermitteln, die Gefäßintegrität vermindern und gleichzeitig vasokonstriktorisch und prothrombotisch wirken.

Das Problem dieses Krankheitsbildes und des geringen Verständnisses seiner Ursachen wird noch deutlicher, wenn man bedenkt, daß die hier kurz angesprochenen Pathomechanismen nicht nur bei inflammatorischen Erkrankungen, sondern auch z. B. bei der Pathogenese der Arteriosklerose erwähnt werden. Ziel des vorliegenden Buches ist es, die Pathogenese der Sepsis – da, wo möglich – krankheitsspezifisch darzustellen, aber gleichzeitig auch noch offene Fragen anzusprechen. Deswegen wurde zunächst die transkriptionelle Aktivierung durch Mediatoren der Sepsis dargestellt und aufgezeigt, daß die Aktivierung von Transkriptionsfaktoren nun auch in vivo am Patienten in klinischen Studien untersucht werden kann.

Ein Zielsystem der transkriptionellen Aktivierung ist die Gerinnung. Deswegen wurde ihr Mechanismus dargestellt und ganz besonders auf die neuen Daten zur Bedeutung der intrinsischen Gerinnung Wert gelegt. Nicht nur der „extrinsisch" aktive Tissue Factor, sondern auch bakterielle Oberflächen können aktiv an der Aktivierung der Gerinnung partizipieren.

Die der Sepsis zugrunde liegenden Erkrankungen sind vielfältig und betreffen alle Disziplinen der Medizin und Intensivmedizin. Von besonderer Bedeutung sind hierbei die entzündlichen Erkrankungen, weswegen die Interaktion des Gerinnungssystems mit der Entzündung dargestellt wurde. Ansätze zur Therapie der Sepsis und der Gerinnungsstörung bei Sepsis wurden im Sinne der „evidence based medicine“ zusammengestellt.

Aber gerade bei der Sepsis hat die „evidence based medicine“ Grenzen. Dies liegt u.a. an der Heterogenität der der Sepsis zugrunde liegenden Erkrankungen, der schwierigen Klassifikation des Krankheitsstadiums und der großen Fallzahlen, die nötig sind, um angesichts dieser nicht kontrollierbaren Variablen aussagefähige Ergebnisse zu erzielen. Die magische Therapie der Sepsis gibt es genauso wenig wie den „typischen“ Sepsis-Patienten. Dies betrifft nicht nur die Störungen der Gerinnung, sondern auch die vaskulären Veränderungen, die Niereninsuffizienz bei Sepsis und die kardialen Komplikationen. Daher wurde die Behandlung dieser Komplikationen der Sepsis so dargestellt, daß dem behandelnden Arzt die Möglichkeit aufgezeigt wird, eine individuell differenzierte Behandlung auszuwählen.

Somit weist dieses Buch dem Kliniker einen Weg von der Pathophysiologie, zur Darstellung der klinischen Symptome, hin zur Behandlung der Sepsis.

Heidelberg und Tübingen, August 1999

E. Martin
P. Nawroth

Inhaltsverzeichnis

Autorenverzeichnis

D'Angelo, A., Dr.
Servizio di Coagulazione, IRCCS H S. Raffaele, Via Olgettina 60, 20132 Milano, Italy

Baudo, F., Dr.
Unita di Emostasi e Trombosi, Divisione di Ematologia, Ospedale Niguarda, Milano, Italy

Bierhaus, A., Dr.
Universitätsklinikum Tübingen, Sektion Vaskuläre Medizin, Medizinische Klinik IV, Otfried-Müller-Str. 10, 72076 Tübingen

Böhrer, H., Prof. Dr.
Klinik für Anästhesiologie, Universität Heidelberg, Im Neuenheimer Feld 110, 69120 Heidelberg, Germany

Caimi, T. M.
Unita' di Emostasi e Trombosi, Divisione di Ematologia, Ospedale Niguarda, Milano, Italy

Caliezi, C., Dr.
Hämatologisches Zentrallabor der Universität, Inselspital, 3010 Bern, Switzerland

Calori, G.
Epidemiology Unit, Ospedale S. Raffaele, Milano, Italy

de Cataldo, F.
Unita di Emostasi e Trombosi, Ospedale Niguarda, Milano, Italy

Della Valle, Patrizia
Servizio di Coagulazione, IRCCS H S. Raffaele, Milano, Italy

Eckardt, K.-U., PD Dr.
Medizinische Klinik mit Schwerpunkt Nephrologie und Intensivmedizin, Charité, Campus Virchow-Klinikum, Augustenburger Platz 1, 13353 Berlin, Germany

Groeneveld, A. B. J., Dr.
Medical Intensive Care Unit, Free University Hospital, De Boelelaan 1117, 1081 HV Amsterdam, The Netherlands

Giudici, Daniela
Unita di Terapia Intensiva, IRCCS H S. Raffaele, Milano, Italy

Hack, C. E., Prof. Dr.
Central Laboratory of the Netherlands Red Cross Blood Transfusion Service and Department of Internal Medicine, Academic Hospital of the Free University Amsterdam, 1006 AK Amsterdam, The Netherlands

Herwald, H., Dr.
Lund University, Department of Cell and Molecular Biology, Section for Molecular Pathogenesis, P.O. Box 94, 221 00 Lund, Sweden

Janssen, R., Dr.
Service de Réanimation Médicale, Hôpital de Hautepierre, Avenue Molière, 67098 Strasbourg Cedex, France

Kemkes-Matthes, B., PD Dr.
Zentrum für Innere Medizin, Klinikstraße 36, 35385 Gießen, Germany

Kurosawa, S.
Cardiovascular Biology Research, Oklahoma Medical Research Foundation, Oklahoma City, OK, USA

Legnani, Cristina
Dipartimento di Angiologia, Ospedale S. Orsola, Bologna, Italy

Mayer, N., Prof. Dr.
Abteilung für Anästhesie und allgemeine Intensivmedizin, Universität Wien, Währinger Gürtel 18–20, 1090 Wien, Austria

Mebazaa, A., Dr.
Département d'Anesthésiologie-Réanimation, Hôpital Lariboisière, 2, rue Ambroise-Paré, 75475 Paris Cedex 10, France

Nawroth, P., Prof. Dr.
Universitätsklinikum Tübingen, Sektion Vaskuläre Medizin, Medizinische Klinik IV und Poliklinik, Otfried-Müller-Str. 10, 72076 Tübingen

Palareti, G., Dr.
Dipartimento di Angiologia, Ospedale S. Orsola, Bologna, Italy

Pneumatikos, I., Dr.
Medical Intensive Care Unit, Free University Hospital, De Boelelaan 1117, 1081 HV Amsterdam, The Netherlands

Ravizza, A., Dr.
Dipartimento di Terapia Intensiva, Ospedale Niguarda, Milano, Italy

Ridolfi, Lorenza, Dr.
Unita di Terapia Intensiva, Ospedale S. Orsola, Bologna, Italy

Schneider, F., Prof. Dr.
Service de Réanimation Médicale, Hôpital de Hautepierre, Avenue Molière, 67098 Strasbourg Cedex, France

Stoclet, J. C., Prof. Dr.
Laboratoire de Pharmacologie et de Physiopathologie cellulaires, URA CNRS 600, Faculté de Pharmacie, 74 route du Rhin, 67401 Illkirch, France

Tempé, J. D., Prof. Dr.
Service de Réanimation Médicale, Hôpital de Hautepierre, Avenue Molière, 67098 Strasbourg Cedex, France

Wallner, T., Prof. Dr.
Abteilung für Anästhesie und allgemeine Intensivmedizin, Universität Wien, Währinger Gürtel 18–20, 1090 Wien, Austria

Wuillemin, W. A., PD Dr. Dr.
Hämatologisches Zentrallabor der Universität, Inselspital, 3010 Bern, Switzerland

Zeerleder, S., Dr.
Hämatologisches Zentrallabor der Universität, Inselspital, 3010 Bern, Switzerland

Die Bedeutung von NF-κB und AP-1 bei der Sepsis

H. Böhrer, A. Bierhaus und P. Nawroth

Transkription und Transkriptionsfaktoren

Transkription und Translation sind Prämissen jeglicher Proteinentstehung, wobei auch die pathologische Überproduktion von pro- bzw. antiinflammatorischen Mediatoren im Rahmen einer Sepsis durch diese Prozesse bedingt ist. Beim ersten Schritt, der Transkription, wird im Zellkern die Information der DNA auf einen mRNA-Strang übertragen, der dann als Grundlage für die Proteinproduktion an den Ribosomen dient [12]. Die Transkription wird durch Transkriptionsfaktoren reguliert, die innerhalb eines Promotorbereiches binden und somit die Expression derjenigen Gene modulieren, die vom Promotor aus kontrolliert werden [10].

Nuclear Factor kappa B (NF-κB) und Activator Protein 1 (AP-1) sind Transkriptionsfaktoren. NF-κB kontrolliert die Transkription einer ganzen Reihe von Genen, die bei Entzündungsprozessen aktiviert werden. Bekannt ist die Bedeutung von NF-κB inzwischen beispielsweise bei entzündlichen Darmerkrankungen [2], bei Asthma bronchiale [8] oder auch bei instabiler Angina pectoris [11]. Weiterhin reguliert NF-κB die Zytokin-Induktion des Gens für die induzierbare NO-Synthase [13]. NF-κB kann in unterschiedlichen Konfigurationen auftreten. Als Prototyp gilt die heterodimere Form bestehend aus einer p50- und einer p65-Untereinheit (Abb. 1). Im inaktiven Zustand ist das Dimer an den zytoplasmatischen Inhibitor IκB gebunden. Bei Aktivierung löst sich IκB vom dimeren Komplex, der in den Zellkern transloziert, dort am entsprechenden Promotorbereich bindet und die Transkription initiiert (Abb. 2).

Der Transkriptionsfaktor AP-1 spielt im Immunsystem ebenfalls eine wichtige Rolle [7]. Auch dieser Transkriptionsfaktor tritt in unterschiedlichen Konfigurationen als Homo- oder Heterodimer auf (s. Abb. 1). Die Jun-Untereinheit kann beispielsweise als c-Jun oder JunD vorliegen, wobei mit c-Fos Heterodimere gebildet werden können. Eine Dimerbildung ist weiterhin mit Untereinheiten von ATF („activating transcription factor") möglich. AP-1 interagiert mit der DNA nach dem Prinzip des Leucin-Reißverschlusses („leucine zipper"), so daß AP-1 zur bZIP-Familie zählt.

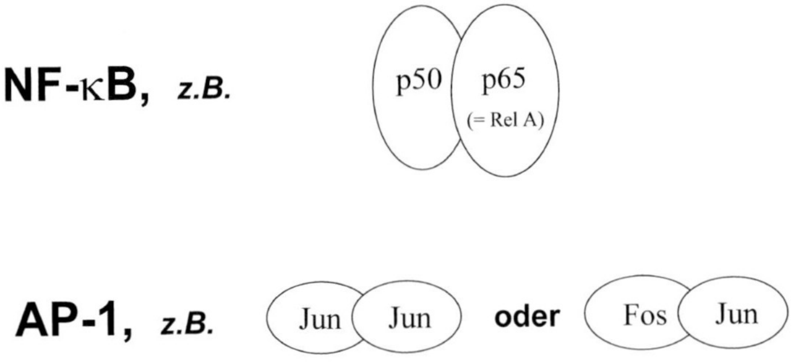

Abb. 1. Die Transkriptionsfaktoren Nuclear Factor kappa B (NF-κB) und Activator Protein 1 (AP-1) können in unterschiedlichen Konfigurationen auftreten. NF-κB kommt in der Regel als heterodimere Form vor, AP-1 kann sowohl als Homo- als auch als Heterodimer vorliegen

Abb. 2. Bei Aktivierung von NF-κB löst sich der zytoplasmatische Inhibitor IκB vom dimeren Komplex, der in den Zellkern transloziert, dort am entsprechenden Promotorbereich bindet und die Transkription initiiert

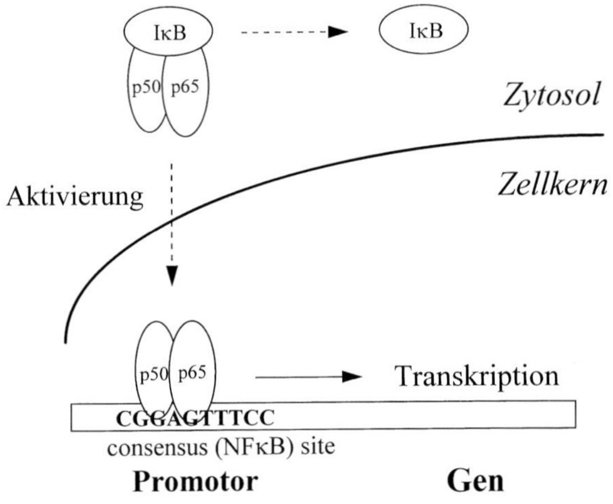

Experimentelles Modell

Zur Klärung der Frage, inwieweit die beiden genannten Transkriptionsfaktoren eine Rolle bei der Sepsis spielen, wurde zuerst ein Tiermodell etabliert. Bei weiblichen BALB/c-Mäusen im Alter von 12 Wochen wurde hierzu ein intravenöser somatischer Gentransfer durchgeführt. Die DNA wurde dabei an Liposomen gebunden in die Schwanzvene injiziert. Die Kontrollgruppe erhielt nur den Expressionsvektor pXT_1, während den beiden anderen Gruppen jeweils IκB als Inhibitor von NF-κB und „mutated Jun“ (mJun) als Inhibitor von AP-1 verabreicht wurde. Nach erfolgtem Gentransfer wurde mit der intraperitonealen Gabe einer Mischung aus 1,75 μg Endotoxin (LPS E. coli 0111 : B4) und D-Galaktosamin eine Sepsis induziert [5].

Ergebnisse

Die Überlebensrate der Tiere betrug 24 Stunden nach Auslösen der Sepsis in der Kontrollgruppe ca. 45%, während in den beiden Gruppen mit Inhibition der Transkriptionsfaktoren die Überlebensrate mit 80% signifikant höher lag (Abb. 3). Somit senkte der intravenöse somatische Gentransfer durch Hemmung der Transkriptionsfaktoren NF-κB und AP-1 die Sepsisletalität im Tiermodell.

In der Kontrollgruppe kam es nach Endotoxingabe in der Niere zu ausgeprägten Fibrinablagerungen, die in den beiden Gruppen mit Überexpression der Inhibitoren IκB und mJun kaum nachweisbar waren. Da solche Endotoxin-bedingten Fibrinablagerungen Ausgangspunkt von Mikrozirkulationsstörungen und somit Grundlage eines Organversagens sein können, kommt ihnen eine große pathogenetische Bedeutung in der Entwicklung des septischen Multiorganversagens zu.

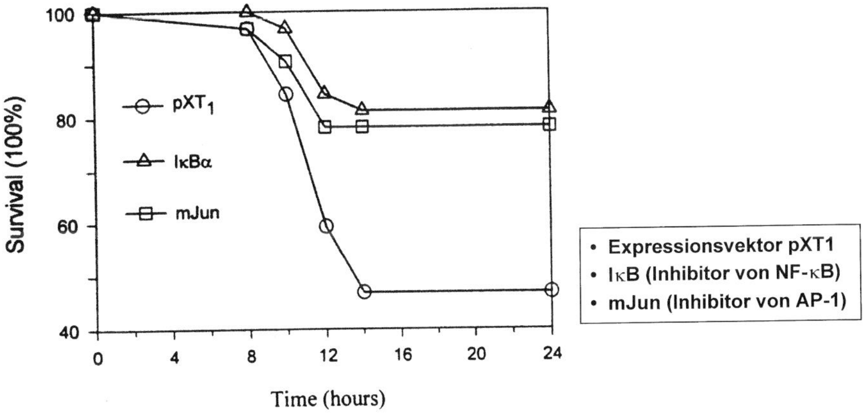

Abb. 3. Effekt eines intravenösen somatischen Gentransfers mit den Inhibitoren IκB und mJun auf die Endotoxin-bedingte Letalität im Mausmodell. Die Gruppe mit dem Expressionsvektor pXT_1 diente als Kontrolle

Bedeutung von Tissue Factor

Die angeführten Fibrinablagerungen reflektieren die Gerinnungsaktivierung in der Sepsis, die über das Extrinsic-System verläuft [3, 9]. Die dominierende Rolle spielt hierbei Tissue Factor (Gewebsthromboplastin), der über einen Tissue-Factor-Faktor-VIIa-Komplex zur Konversion von Faktor X zu Xa führt. Da bekannt ist, daß das Tissue-Factor-Gen unter anderem über eine NFκB- und zwei AP-1-Bindungsstellen transkriptionell reguliert wird [4], lag es nahe, die Bedeutung von Tissue Factor näher zu charakterisieren. Durch Färbung mittels Antikörper gegen Tissue Factor ließ sich nachweisen, daß die Tissue-Factor-Antigen-Expression in der IκB- und mJun-Gruppe nach Endotoxingabe im Vergleich zur Endotoxin-stimulierten Kontrollgruppe deutlich reduziert war. Mit Hilfe der Luciferase-Bestimmung ließ sich zeigen, daß die Aktivität des Tissue-Factor-Promotors nur in der Endotoxin-stimulierten Kontrollgruppe, jedoch nicht in den IκB- und mJun-Gruppen erhöht war (Abb. 4). Somit reduziert die Hemmung der beiden Transkriptionsfaktoren NF-κB und AP-1 die Endotoxin-bedingte Tissue-Factor-Expression.

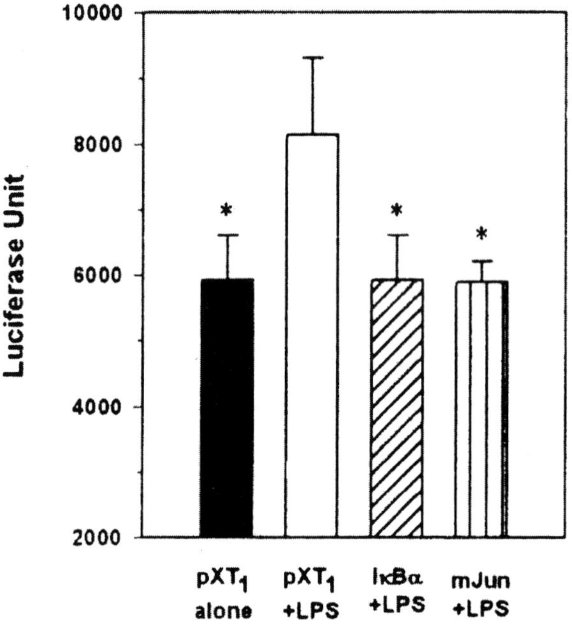

Abb. 4. Erfassung der Aktivität des Tissue-Factor-Promotors mittels Luciferase-Bestimmung nach Gentransfer mit IκB und mJun (und Endotoxin-Stimulation)

Patientenbefunde

Zur klinischen Evaluierung dieser Befunde wurden in die Studie Intensivpatienten einbezogen, welche die Sepsiskriterien der amerikanischen Konsensuskonferenz aus dem Jahre 1991 erfüllten [1]. Der Schweregrad der Erkrankung, der anhand des APACHE-II-Scores quantifiziert wurde, korrelierte gut mit der Bindungsaktivität der Transkriptionsfaktoren (Abb. 5). Insbesondere der Verlauf der NF-κB-Bindungsaktivität erwies sich als Prädiktor für das Überleben bzw. Nicht-Überleben des Patienten. Die Abb. 6 zeigt die hohe NF-κB-Bindungsaktivität im Electrophoretic Mobility Shift Assay bei einem Nicht-Überlebenden im Vergleich zu einem überlebenden, septischen Intensivpatienten.

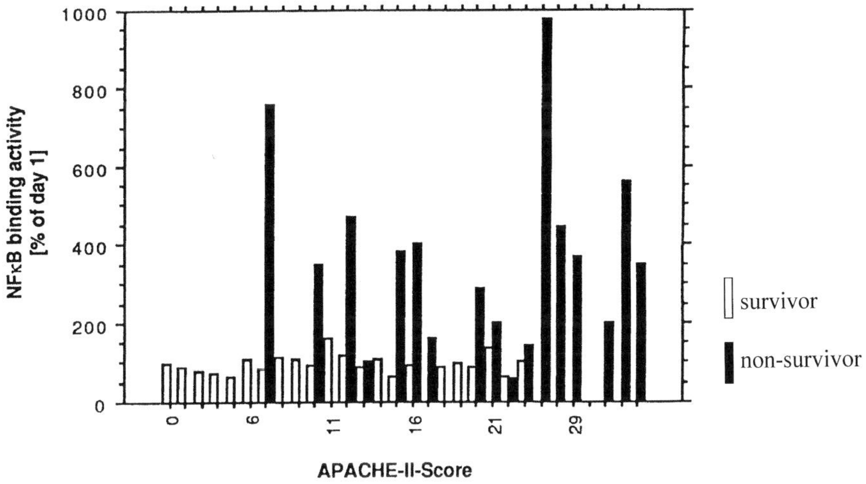

Abb. 5. Korrelation der NF-κB-Bindungsaktivität und APACHE-II-Score bei septischen Intensivpatienten

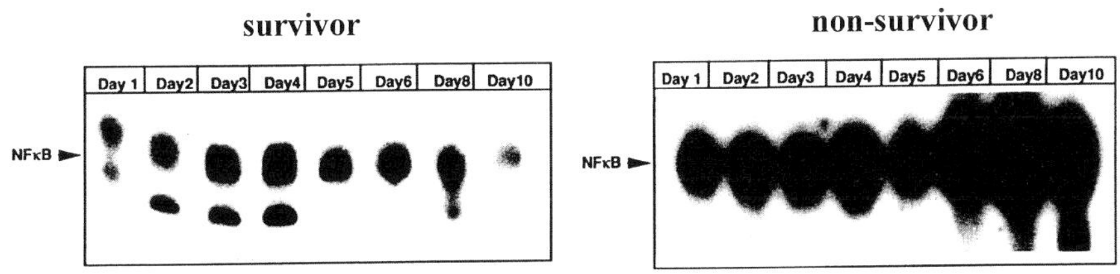

Abb. 6. Beispiel der hohen NF-κB-Bindungsaktivität bei einem Nicht-Überlebenden im Electrophoretic Mobility Shift Assay (im Vergleich zu einem überlebenden, septischen Intensivpatienten)

Schlußfolgerung

Wir schließen aus unseren Befunden, daß die beiden Transkriptionsfaktoren NF-κB und AP-1 eine wichtige Rolle in der Sepsis spielen. Dies gilt sowohl für die tierexperimentelle Situation der Endotoxin-induzierten Sepsis als auch für den septischen Intensivpatienten. Insbesondere die Beeinflussung von NF-κB könnte eine zukünftige therapeutische Modalität darstellen [6].

Literatur

1. American College of Chest Physicians/Society of Critical Care Medicine Consensus Conference (1992) Definitons for sepsis and organ failure and guidelines for the use of innovative therapies in sepsis. Crit Care Med 20:864–874
2. Barnes PJ, Karin M (1997) Nuclear factor-κB – a pivotal transcription factor in chronic inflammatory diseases. N Engl J Med 336:1066–1071
3. Biemond BJ, Levi M, ten Cate H et al. (1995) Complete inhibition of endotoxin-induced coagulation activation in chimpanzees with a monoclonal Fab fragment against factor VII/VIIa. Thromb Haemost 73:223–230
4. Bierhaus A, Zhang Y, Deng Y et al. (1995) Mechanism of the tumor necrosis factor alpha-mediated induction of endothelial tissue factor. J Biol Chem 270:26419–26432
5. Böhrer H, Qiu F, Zimmermann T, et al. (1997) Role of NFκB in the mortality of sepsis. J Clin Invest 100:972–985
6. Böhrer H, Nawroth PP (1998) Nuclear factor κB – a new therapeutic approach? (Editorial) Intensive Care Med 24:1129–1130
7. Foletta VC, Segal DH, Cohen DR (1998) Transcriptional regulation in the immune system: all roads lead to AP-1. J Leukoc Biol 63:139–152
8. Hart LA, Krishnan VL, Adcock IM, Barnes PJ, Chung KF (1998) Activation on localization of transcription factor, nuclear factor-κB, in asthma. Am J Respir Crit Care Med 158:1585–1592
9. Levi M, ten Cate H, Bauer KA et al. (1994) Inhibition of endotoxin-induced activation of coagulation and fibrinolysis by pentoxifylline or by a monoclonal anti-tissue factor antibody in chimpanzees. J Clin Invest 93:114–120
10. Papavassiliou AG (1995) Transcription factors. N Engl J Med 332:45–47
11. Ritchie ME (1998) Nuclear factor-κB is selectively and markedly activated in humans with unstable angina pectoris. Circulation 98:1707–1713
12. Rosenthal N (1994) DNA and the genetic code. N Engl J Med 331:39–41
13. Taylor BS, de Vera ME, Ganster RW et al. (1998) Multiple NF-kappaB enhancer elements regulate cytokine induction of the human inducible nitric oxide synthase gene. J Biol Chem 273:15148–15156

KAPITEL 2

Aktivierung der Gerinnung bei Sepsis

B. Kemkes-Matthes

Einleitung

Die Sepsis ist auch heute, trotz intensivmedizinischer Behandlung und erheblich verbesserter Antibiotikatherapie, ein äußerst bedrohliches Krankheitsbild. Inzidenz und Mortalität haben sich in den letzten Jahren kaum geändert.

Die betroffenen Patienten versterben im allgemeinen nicht an der primären Infektion, sondern meist an durch Folgekomplikationen bedingtem Multiorganversagen.

Unter diesen Folgekomplikationen nimmt die Verbrauchskoagulopathie, in deren Verlauf es zu Thrombosierung, Organversagen und schließlich zu Blutungen kommt, einen zentralen Stellenwert ein.

Definition

Unter Sepsis versteht man komplexe Reaktionen des Körpers auf eingeschwemmte Mikroorganismen bzw. deren Toxine. Meist handelt es sich um gramnegative, seltener um grampositive Bakterien, Pilze oder Parasiten. Die Infektion kann „direkt", z. B. durch Keimeinschwemmung im Rahmen von Verletzungen, oder auch „indirekt", z. B. durch Keimübertritt aus dem Darm im Rahmen von Schockzuständen, zustande kommen.

Da bei Patienten mit schweren septischen Krankheitsbildern Keime häufig nicht nachweisbar sind, wurde in den letzten Jahren versucht, das Krankheitsbild der Sepsis neu zu definieren. Dazu wurden sog. ***„Sepsis-Kriterien"*** aufgestellt:

- Temperatur >38 °C oder <36 °C
- Herzfrequenz >90/min
- Respiratorische Insuffizienz: Tachypnoe >20 Atemzüge/min bzw. $PaCO_2$ <32 mmHg
- Leukozytose >12 000/ul
- Leukopenie <4000/ul

Um die Diagnose „Sepsis“ zu stellen, genügt der Keimnachweis plus Erfüllung von 2 Sepsis-Kriterien. Bei der ***„schweren Sepsis“*** kommt es zusätzlich zur Organdysfunktion, beim ***„septischen Schock“*** darüber hinaus zum Blutdruckabfall mit systolischen Werten unter 90 mmHg. Als schwerste Form der Sepsis wird das ***SIRS*** – das „systemic inflammatory response syndrome“ – angesehen, dabei sind typischerweise keine Keime nachweisbar.

Gerinnungsveränderungen bei Sepsis

Im Rahmen septischer Erkrankungen kommt es immer zu Gerinnungsveränderungen im Sinne der ***Gerinnungsaktivierung:*** Eindringende Mikroorganismen bewirken Aktivierung des Monozyten-Makrophagen-Systems, in der Folge kommt es zur Freisetzung inflammatorischer Zytokine wie IL-1β, IL-6 und TNFα sowie zur Expression von Tissue Factor (Abb. 1). Die Expression von Tissue Factor und damit die Aktivierung des extrinsischen Gerinnungssystems scheint der Haupttrigger-Mechanismus für die Aktivierung des (extrinsischen) Gerinnungssystems bei Sepsis zu sein. Die Tissue-Factor-Expression erfolgt sowohl monozytär als auch über Zytokin-stimuliertes Endothel. Am Endothel kommt es darüber hinaus zur Downregulation von Thrombomodulin, vermehrter Expression von Plasminogen-Aktivator-Inhibitor (PAI) und Adhäsionsmolekülen – in der Summe also zur Ausprägung der „thrombogenen“ Endotheloberfläche.

Das beschriebene „Ankurbeln“ der Gerinnungskaskade bei Sepsis induziert Gerinnungsaktivierung, welche durch die „thrombogene“ Endotheloberfläche noch aggraviert wird.

Abb. 1. Gerinnungsaktivierung bei Sepsis

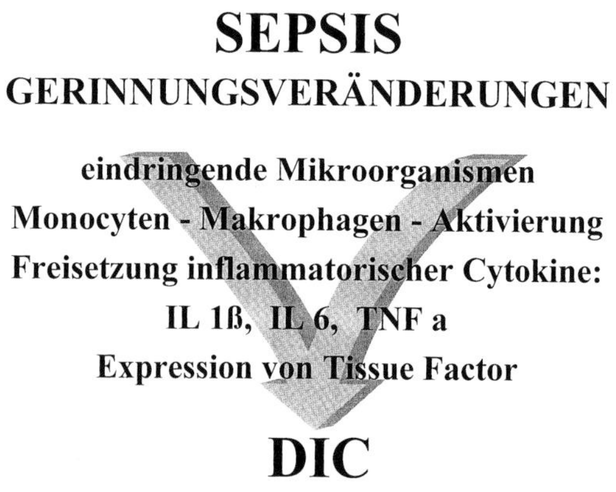
SEPSIS
GERINNUNGSVERÄNDERUNGEN
eindringende Mikroorganismen
Monocyten - Makrophagen - Aktivierung
Freisetzung inflammatorischer Cytokine:
IL 1ß, IL 6, TNF a
Expression von Tissue Factor
DIC

Die Aktivierung des Gerinnungssystems bei Sepsis kann sich in extrem unterschiedlicher Ausprägung äußern: In den blandesten Fällen kommt es lediglich zum Nachweis von Gerinnungsaktivierungsmarkern wie Prothrombin Fragment F 1+2, TAT-Komplexen und D-Dimer, in den schwersten Fällen zum Vollbild der Verbrauchskoagulopathie mit Abfall von Gerinnungsfaktoren, -inhibitoren und Thrombozyten.

Aus einer Einzeluntersuchung kann die Diagnose der Verbrauchskoagulopathie im allgemeinen nicht gestellt werden, da zur Diagnosestellung insbesondere der Verlauf der einzelnen Parameter wichtig ist.

Klassisch ist die Verminderung von Quick-Wert und die Verlängerung der PTT als Ausdruck des durch den Verbrauch verminderten prokoagulatorischen Potentials. Darüber hinaus sind charakteristisch die Abnahme von Antithrombin, aber auch von anderen Inhibitoren wie Protein C und S, als Ausdruck des erhöhten Umsatzes des Inhibitorpotentials sowie ein progredienter Abfall der Thrombozyten (Abb. 2). Fibrinogen, welches bei septischen Erkrankungen im Rahmen der Akutphasenreaktion meist zunächst hochreguliert ist, kann, auch wenn die übrigen Gerinnungs-Parameter bereits pathologisch sind, noch im Normbereich liegen, zeigt aber immer abfallende Tendenz.

Sowohl für die Diagnosestellung als auch für die Verlaufskontrolle der Verbrauchskoagulopathie sind engmaschige Messungen von Quick-Wert, PTT, Antithrombin, Fibrinogen und Thrombozyten essentiell. Gerinnungsaktivierungsparameter wie Prothrombin Fragment F 1+2, TAT-Komplexe, oder D-Dimer als Ausdruck der reaktiven Fibrinolyse können in der Frühphase der Gerinnungsaktivierung wichtige Hinweise liefern. Für die Beurteilung des Vollbildes der Verbrauchskoagulopathie sind diese Parameter nicht (mehr) notwendig.

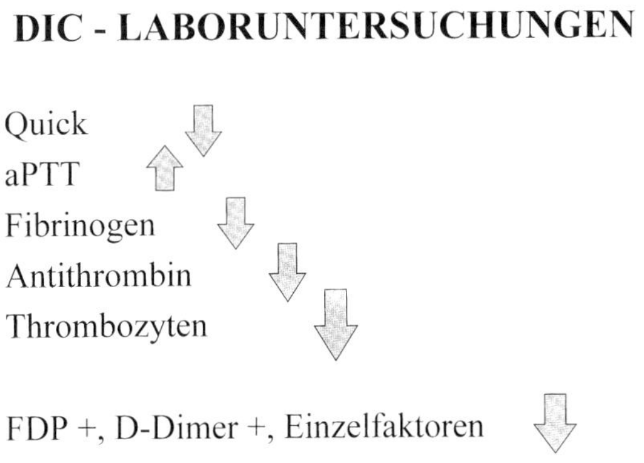

Abb. 2. Veränderungen von Gerinnungsparametern bei Patienten mit Sepsis

Klinik der Verbrauchskoagulopathie

Die Sepsis ist die häufigste Ursache der Verbrauchskoagulopathie. Dabei steht das septische Geschehen klinisch zunächst im Vordergrund. Mit zunehmender Gerinnungsaktivierung kann sich die Verbrauchsrekation jedoch verselbständigen und klinisch führend werden: Es kommt zur Ausbildung von Mikro- selten auch von Makro-Thrombosen, welche zum einen Organversagen induzieren können, zum anderen den weiteren Verbrauch von Gerinnungsfaktoren, -inhibitoren und Thrombozyten triggern, so daß – wenn das Hämostasepotential weitgehend aufgebraucht ist – eine Blutungsneigung resultiert (Abb. 3). Das klassische klinische Bild der Verbrauchskoagulopathie ist daher das gleichzeitige Vorliegen von Thrombose, Blutung und Organversagen.

Abb. 3. Pathophysiologie der Verbrauchskoagulopathie

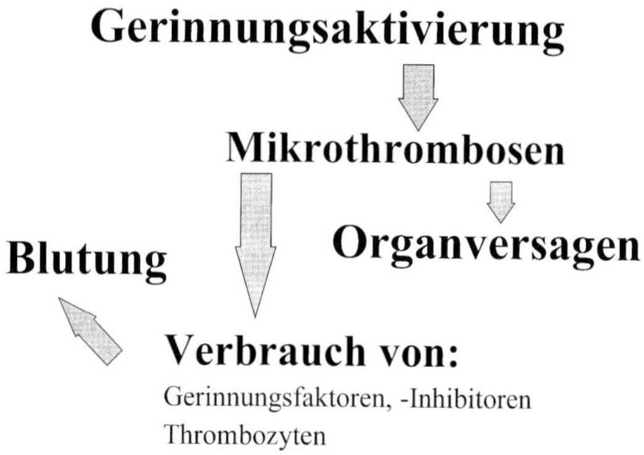

Literatur

1. Dickneite G (1998) Antithrombin III in animal models of sepsis and organ failure. Sem Thromb Hemostas 24 (1): 61–69
2. Kirchmaier CM (1995) Ätiologie und Pathophysiologie der disseminierten intravasalen Gerinnnung. Hämostaseologie 15: 69–78
3. Okajima K (1997) Antithrombin III bei schwerer Sepsis – Antikoagulation und Antiinflammation. Die gelben Hefte 37: 49–54
4. Okajima K, Uchiba M (1998) The anti-inflammatory properties of Antithrombin III: New therapeutic implications. Sem Thromb Hemostas 24 (1): 27–32
5. Ritthaler U, Böhrer H, Nawroth PP (1996) Schwere Sepsis und septischer Schock. Krankenhaus Arzt 69: 512–519
6. Seitz R, Egbring R (1995) Diagnostische Kriterien der disseminierten intravasalen Gerinnung. Hämostaseologie 15: 65–68
7. Vervloet MG, Lambertus GT, Hack GE (1998) Derangements of coagulation and fibrinolysis in critically ill patients with sepsis and septic shock. Sem Thromb Hemostas 24 (1): 33–44

Aktivierung der intrinsischen Gerinnung auf bakteriellen Oberflächen

H. Herwald

Fieber, Hypotonie und Gerinnungsstörungen sind häufig diagnostizierte Symptome bei schwerwiegenden Infektionskrankheiten. Klinische Studien zeigen, daß die Aktivierung des Kontaktphasensystems, das entzündungs- und gerinnungsstimulierende Reaktionen hervorruft, zu diesen Komplikationen beiträgt [1]. Die zugrunde liegenden molekularen Mechanismen sind jedoch noch weitgehend unverstanden. Der vorliegende Beitrag gibt eine kurze Übersicht über neue Untersuchungen, die zeigen, daß das Kontaktphasensystem auf den Oberflächen von Bakterien aktiviert werden kann und welche Folgereaktionen dadurch ausgelöst werden können.

Aktivierung des Kontaktphasensystems

Das Endothel, die Grenzschicht zwischen dem zirkulierenden Blut und dem umgebenden Gewebe, übt wichtige Funktionen in der Kontrolle von Hämostase und Entzündungsvorgängen aus [2]. Stimulierung oder Beschädigung des Endothels führen zu einer Reihe von Folgeerscheinungen, die unter anderem die Regulierung des Blutdruckes, die Freisetzung prokoagulatorischer Substanzen und die Erhöhung der vaskulären Permeabilität beeinflussen können [2]. Diese Effekte lassen sich häufig auf die Aktivierung von endothelial regulierten Effektorsystemen zurückführen. Das Kontaktphasensystem gehört zu dieser Gruppe von regulatorischen Kaskaden und kann nach Stimulierung koagulative und inflammatorische Reaktionen induzieren [3]. Es besteht aus den drei Serinproteasen Faktor XII, Faktor XI und Plasma Kallikrein (F XII, F XI, PK) sowie dem Hilfsfaktor hochmolekulares Kininogen (HK) [4].

Die Wechselwirkungen von Kontaktphasenfaktoren mit zellulären Oberflächenstrukturen können zur Aktivierung des Systems führen. Daneben sind negativ geladenen Materialien, wie zum Beispiel Glas oder Kaolin, in der Lage, die Aktivierung zu initiieren. Auf zellulärer Ebene wurden hauptsächlich die Interaktionen von Kontaktphasenfaktoren mit Endothelzellen, Neutrophilen und Thrombozyten untersucht [5–9]; die molekularen Mechanismen der Aktivierung auf diesen Zellen konnten allerdings noch nicht vollständig aufgeklärt werden. Dagegen ist der Mechanismus auf negativ geladenen synthetischen Oberflächen besser verstanden. So zeigen In-vitro-Studien, daß die Initiierung des Kontaktphasensystems durch die partielle Aktivierung von oberflächengebundenem F XII (F XIIa) ausgelöst wird. Anschließend kommt es zu einer

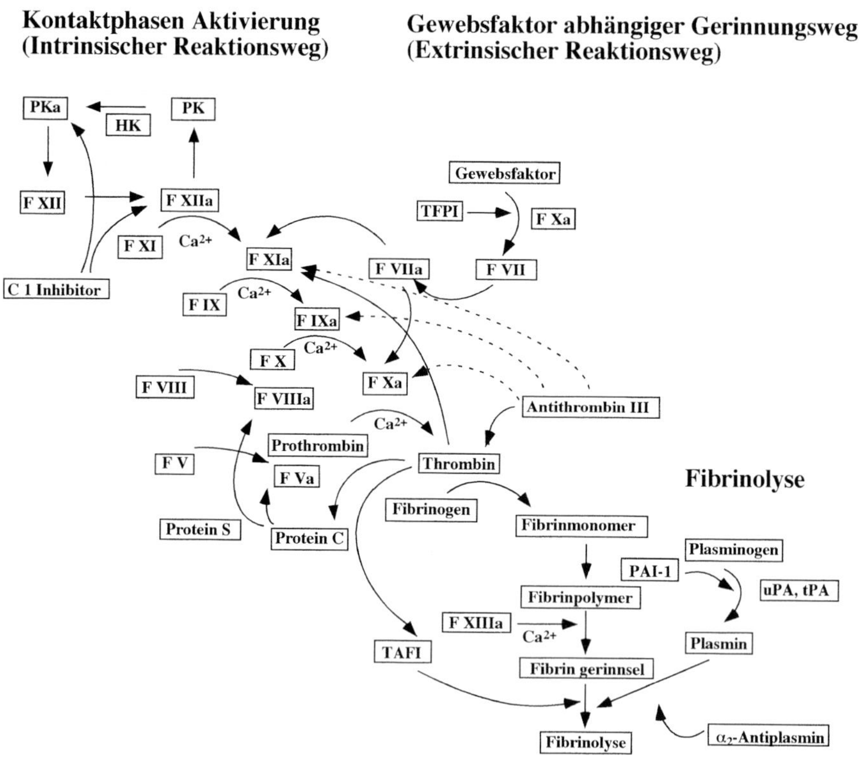

Abb. 1. Die Blutgerinnungskaskade beim Menschen. Die Gerinnungskaskade ist in einen intrinsischen und extrinsischen Reaktionsweg unterteilt. Proteine, die in Gerinnung partizipieren, sind aufgrund ihrer Funktion unterteilt in: Serinproteasen (F VII, F IX, F X, F XI, F XII, PK, Plasminogen, Prothrombin), Hilfsfaktoren (F V, F VIII, Gewebsfaktor, Protein S) und Proteaseninhibitoren (α_2-Antiplasmin, Antithrombin III, C1 Inhibitor, PAI-1, Protein C, TAFI, TFPI). Proteine nach ihrer Aktivierung sind mit „a" gekennzeichnet. Pfeile symbolisieren die proteolytische Umwandlung. Folgende Abkürzungen wurden verwendet: *F*, Faktor; *HK*, Hochmolekulares Kininogen; *PK*, Plasmakallikrein; *TAFI*, Thrombin Activatable Fibrinolysis Inhibitor; *TFPI*, Tissue Factor Pathway Inhibitor; *tPA*, Tissue Plasminogen Activator und *uPA*, Urokinase-Type Plasminogen Activator

Aktivierung von PK (PKa) durch F XIIa [10]. PKa hat zwei Funktionen: Zum einen induziert es eine Erhöhung der proteolytischen Aktivität von F XIIa, wodurch im folgenden die Umwandlung von F XI in die aktive Form (F Xla) und somit die Initiierung der Gerinnungskaskade ermöglicht werden (Abb. 1). Zum anderen spaltet PKa HK unter Freisetzung von Bradykinin. Bradykinin gehört zur Familie der Kinine und ruft eine Reihe von Entzündungsreaktionen, wie Schmerz, Ödembildung und Erhöhung der vaskulären Permeabiltiät, hervor [11].

Die Aktivierung des Kontaktphasensystems bei Infektionskrankheiten

Zahlreiche Studien aus den letzten dreißig Jahre belegen, daß die massive Aktivierung des Kontaktphasensystems bei Infektionskrankheiten zu lebensbedrohlichen Komplikationen führen kann [12]. So berichten bereits Studien aus den 70er Jahren, daß die Plasmakonzentrationen von Kontaktphasenproteinen bei Patienten mit hypotoner Sepsis deutlich unterhalb der normalen Werte liegen [13]. Neuere Untersuchungen zeigen, daß eine drastische Reduktion der Konzentrationen an F XII und HK im Blut von Patienten mit SIRS (Systemic Inflammatory Response Syndrome) mit einem tödlichen Ausgang der Krankheit korreliert [14].

Im Laufe der letzten Jahrzehnte sind eine Reihe bakteriell sekretierter Substanzen identifiziert und charakterisiert worden, dic zu einer Aktivierung des Systems führen können. Der wohl seit längstem bekannte Stimulator des Kontaktphasensystems, Endotoxin oder LPS, ist ein potenter Aktivator von F XII [15]. Darüber hinaus können geringe Dosen an LPS auch zu einer Kontaktphasen-unabhängigen Aktivierung von F XI führen [16]. Ferner sind in den letzten Jahren eine Reihe von Proteasen isoliert worden, die in der Lage sind, das System zu initiieren [17–23]. Interessanterweise benutzen die Bakterien unterschiedliche Mechanismen, um Kinine zu generieren. Während einige Proteasen Kininogene unter Freisetzung von physiologisch aktiven Kininen spalten, aktivieren andere F XII oder PK und induzieren somit indirekt die Kininfreisetzung (Tabelle 1). Da Kinine eine Erhöhung der vaskulären Permeabilität induzieren, könnte durch das Ausschütten dieser Hormone eine effiziente Ausbreitung des Pathogens im Wirtsorganismus ermöglicht werden.

Neben eukaryontischen Zelloberflächen und negativ geladenen synthetischen Materialien exponieren auch bakterielle Zellwandbestandteile geeignete Strukturen, die Kontaktphasenproteine assemblieren und deren Aktivierung

Tabelle 1. Aktivierung des Kontaktphasensystems durch bakterielle Proteasen

Mikroorganismus	Zielprotein	Referenz
Aspergillus melleus	F XII	[17]
Bacillus stearothermophilus	F XII/PK	[17]
Bacillus subtilis	F XII/PK	[17]
Porphyromonas gingivalis	HK	[22]
Porphyromonas gingivalis	PK	[21]
Porphyromonas gingivalis	PK/HK	[35]
Pseudomonas aeruginosa	F XII	[17]
Pseudomonas aeruginosa	nicht bekannt	[18]
Serratia marcescens	F XII	[17]
Staphylococcus aureus	HK	[17]
Streptococcus pyogenes	HK	[23]
Streptomyces caespitosus	HK	[17]
Vibrio cholerae	nicht bekannt	[36]
Vibrio vulnificus	PK	[37]
Vibrio vulnificus	F XII/PK	[17]

induzieren. So zeigte die Untersuchung klinischer Isolate von Sepsispatienten, daß Bakterien der Art *Streptococcus pyogenes*, *Escherichia coli* und *Salmonella* spp. eine hohe Affinität zu HK besitzen (Abb. 2) [24–26]. Eine detailliertere Analyse der Interaktionen von HK mit *E. coli*-Stämmen, isoliert von Patienten mit Sepsis oder gastrointestinalen Infektionen, ergab, daß hauptsächlich enterohämorrhagische, enterotoxische und Sepsis-Stämme HK binden (Abb. 3) [25].

Die Aktivierung des Kontaktphasensystems auf der Oberfläche von *Streptococcus pyogenes*

Die Aktivierung des Kontaktphasensystems durch *Streptococcus pyogenes* wurde erstmals 1991 beschrieben [27]. Diese Studien zeigen, daß die Injektion von bakteriellen Zellwand-assozierten Peptidoglykanen in Ratten zu einer Kontaktphasenaktivierung führt und dies möglicherweise eine wichtige Rolle bei rheumatoider Arthritis spielt [27]. Untersuchungen der molekularen Mechanismen der Kontaktphasenaktivierung auf Streptokokken ergaben, daß bakteriell gebundenes HK proteolytisch gespalten wird. Die dabei entstehenden Degradationsprodukte weisen ein typisches Muster auf, das auf die Freisetzung von Bradykinin durch PKa hindeutet [28]. Diese Vermutung wird durch weitere Un-

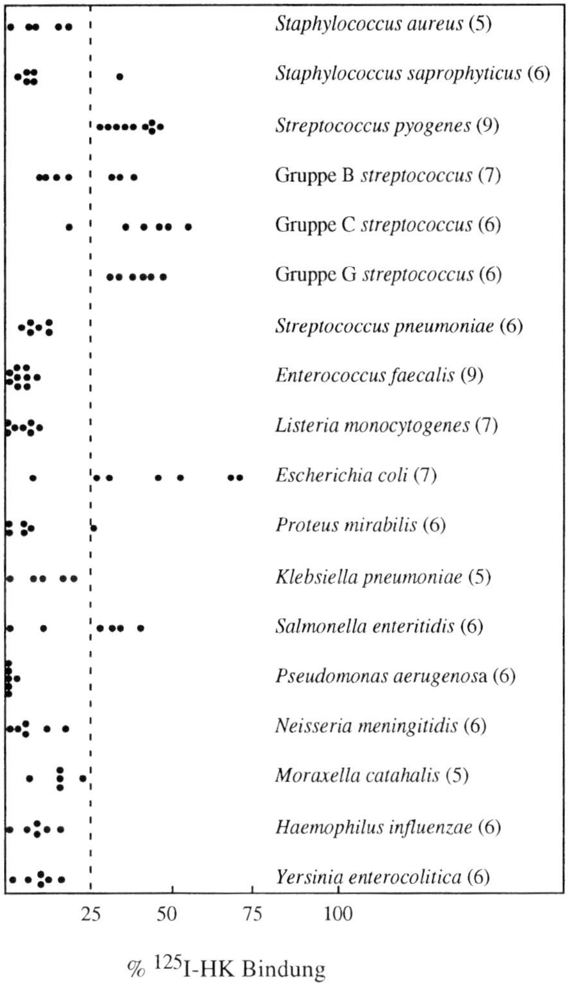

Abb. 2. Bindung von HK an klinischen Isolaten von Sepsispatienten. Die Bindung von HK an 118 bakterielle Stämme (18 verschiedene Arten) von Sepsispatienten wurde untersucht

tersuchungen gestützt, die zeigen, daß die Inkubation von Plasma mit Streptokokken und der anschließenden Behandlung mit PKa zu einer Erhöhung der Bradykinin-Konzentration im Überstand führen [28]. Die Ergebnisse implizieren, daß das Kontaktphasensystem endogen und ohne Hilfe bakterieller Zellwand-assozierter Proteasen initiiert wird. Die Streptokokken-induzierte Kontaktphasenaktivierung scheint somit nach einem analogen Mechanismus zu verlaufen, wie für negativ geladene artifizielle Oberflächen beschrieben [28].

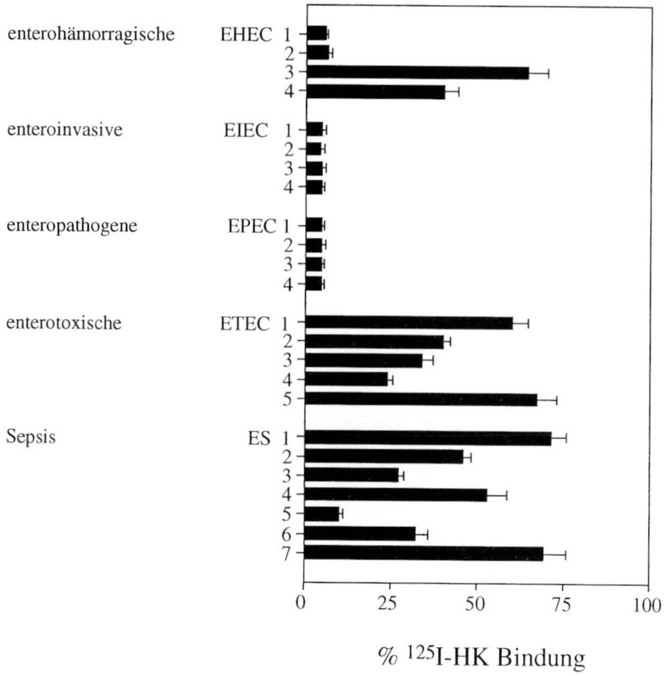

Abb. 3. Bindung von HK an pathogene *E. coli*-Stämme. Die Bindung von HK an 24 *E. coli*-Stämme von Patienten mit Sepsis oder gastrointestinalen Infektionen wurde analysiert

Die Aktivierung des Kontaktphasensystems auf der Oberfläche gramnegativer Bakterien

Adhärens ist eine wichtige Voraussetzung für pathogene Bakterien, effizient Wirtsgewebe zu kolonisieren. Praktisch alle bekannten virulenten Mikroorganismen exprimieren ein oder mehrere Adhäsionsfaktoren auf ihren Oberflächen, wie zum Beispiel Fimbrien oder Pili. Gewöhnlich liegen die Gene, die für die Synthese von Adhäsionsfaktoren verantwortlich sind, auf Pathogenitätsinseln im Chromosom oder auf Plasmiden. Bakterielle Adhäsine verschiedener Arten oder Serotypen besitzen charakteristische immunogene und adhäsive Eigenschaften, die ihre Infektionsroute und ihre ökologische Nische im Wirt widerspiegeln. Die unterschiedlichen Klassen von Virulenzfaktoren lassen sich nur schlecht bezüglich ihres phylogenetischen Stammbaumes einteilen, da artverwandte Stämme nicht notwendigerweise ähnliche pathogene Eigenschaften besitzen und daher andere Virulenzfaktoren benötigen. Gegen Ende der 80er

Jahre wurde eine neue Art von Oberflächenorganelle, im weiteren als „Curli-Organelle" bezeichnet, aus *E. coli* und *Salmonella* spp. isoliert [29,30]. Im Gegensatz zu anderen Adhäsinen sind die Gene, die für Curli kodieren, innerhalb der unterschiedlichen Stämme stark konserviert und in fast allen *E. coli*- und *Salmonella*-Stämmen vorhanden. Das ubiquitäre Auffinden dieser Gene in *E. coli* und *Salmonella* spp. impliziert daher eine wichtige Funktion dieser Organellen als Adhäsionsfaktoren.

Curli-Organellen bestehen aus einer Vielzahl von Proteinuntereinheiten, die in Bündeln auf der bakteriellen Oberfläche aggregieren (Abb. 4). Sie besitzen eine hohe Affinität zu einer Reihe von Zellmembran-, Zellmatrix- und Plasma-Proteinen, wie zum Beispiel zu MHC-Klasse-1-Antigen, Fibronektin oder Plasminogen [31–34]. Neben diesen Proteinen binden Curli-Organellen auch die Kontaktphasenfaktoren und Fibrinogen [25, 26].

Die Assemblierung von Kontaktphasenfaktoren auf Bakterien, die Curli-Organellen exprimieren, führt zu einer erhöhten proteolytischen Aktivität der

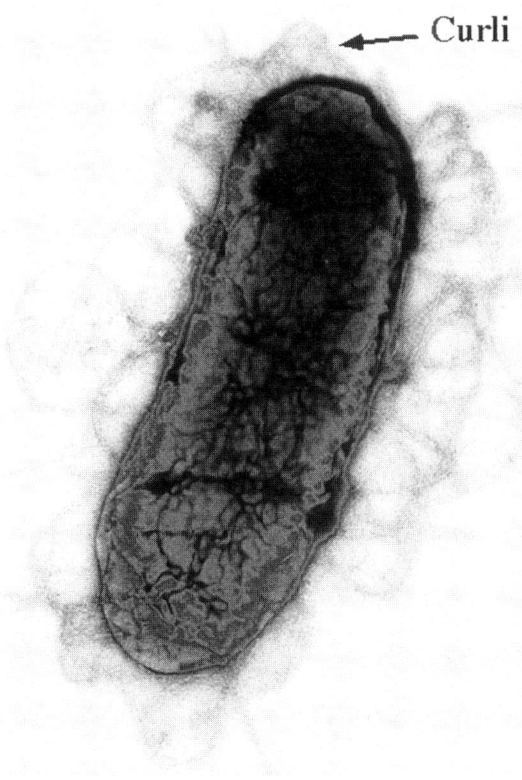

Abb. 4. Elektronenmikroskopische Aufnahme eines Curli-exprimierenden Bakteriums

Abb. 5. Freisetzung von Bradykinin auf bakteriellen Oberflächen. Die Konzentrationen von Bradykinin im Überstand von Curli-exprimierenden *S. typhimurium* und *E. coli*-Bakterien, die mit Plasma präinkubiert wurden, wurde bestimmt. Als Negativkontrolle dienten isogene *S. typhimurium*- und *E. coli*-Mutanten, die kein Curli produzieren

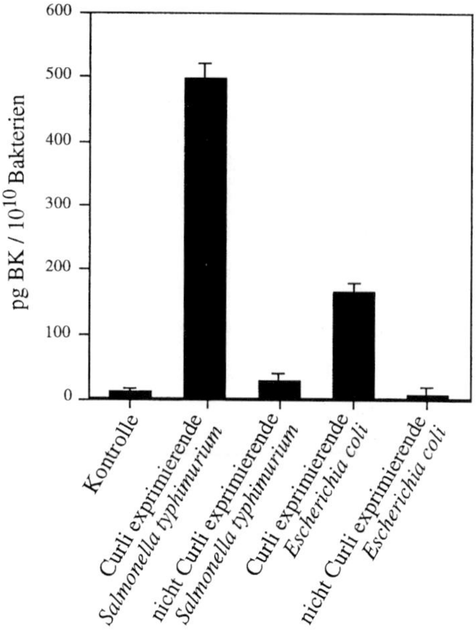

Faktoren und resultiert in der Freisetzung von Bradykinin (Abb. 5). Zudem erzeugt die Absorption von Gerinnungsfaktoren einen hypokoagulativen Zustand, wie die Analyse von Blutproben von Mäusen, die mit Curli-exprimierenden Bakterien infiziert wurden, ergab [26]. Die elektronenmikroskopische Untersuchung der Blutgerinnsel infizierter Mäuse zeigte außerdem, daß die entstandenen Gerinnsel nur aus präzipitierten Erythrozyten bestanden, denen ein Fibrinnetzwerk fehlte und in die Bakterien inkorporiert waren (Abb. 6).

Diese Studien zeigen, daß aktive Kinine an Infektionsherden lokal produziert werden können. Als Folge der Freisetzung kann es zu einer Erhöhung der vaskulären Permeabilität und zu einem Austritt von Plasmabestandteilen in das umgebende Gewebe kommen. Die bakteriell induzierte Bradykinin-Freisetzung kann zwei Vorteile für die Bakterien haben. Zum einen versorgen die in das Gewebe eindringenden Plasmabestandteile Bakterien mit Nährstoffen; zum anderen wäre der Austritt von Bakterien vom Plasma ins Gewebe oder umgekehrt ermöglicht. Verminderte Gerinnbarkeit würde zudem verhindern, daß der Pathogen in einem Fibrinnetzwerk gefangen wird und phagozytierenden Zellen präsentiert werden kann.

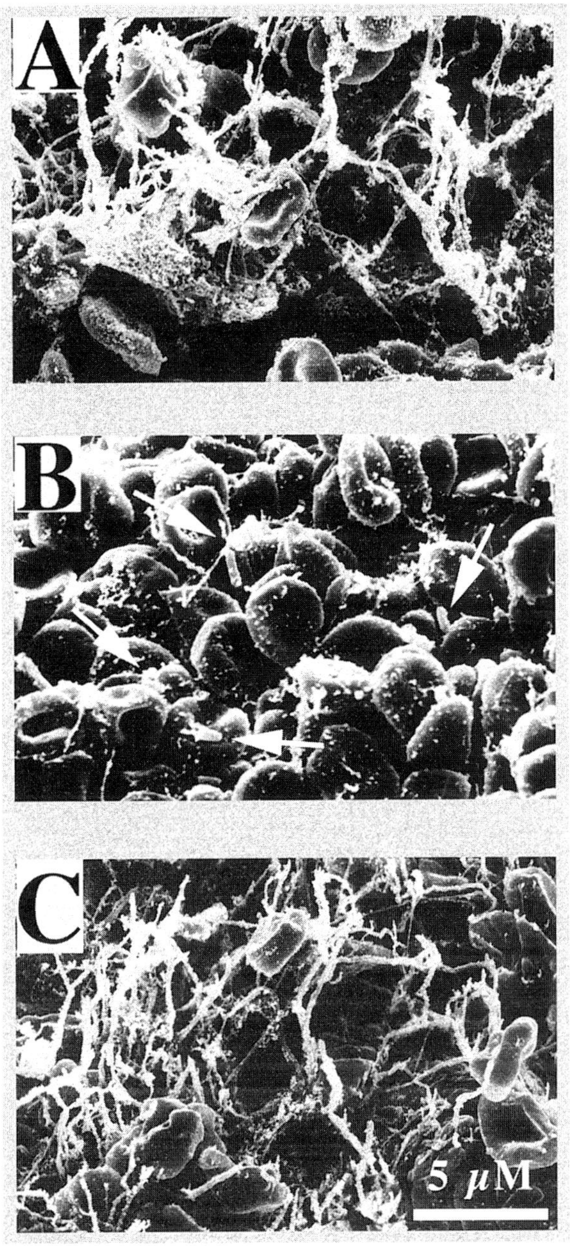

Abb. 6 A–C. Elektronenmikroskopische Aufnahmen von Blutgerinnseln infizierter Mäuse. **A** Kontrollgerinnsel, von einer nicht infizierten Maus; **B** Gerinnsel einer Maus, die mit Curli-produzierenden *E. coli*-Bakterien infiziert wurde; **C** Gerinnsel einer Maus, die mit einer *E. coli*-Mutanten infiziert wurde, die kein Curli exprimiert. *Pfeile* zeigen auf Bakterien im Gerinnsel. Der Balken entspricht 5 μm

Schlußbemerkung

Das Rekrutieren von Wirtsproteinen und die Aktivierung ihrer Effektorsysteme ist ein von pathogenen Bakterien häufig praktizierter Mechanismus, der inflammatorische Reaktionen hervorruft. Die Identifizierung solcher Gast-Wirt-Wechselwirkungen ist eine wichtige Grundlage, um neue antibakterielle Konzepte zu entwickeln. Medikamente, die eine Stimulierung von wirtseigenen Effektorsystemen durch Mikroorganismen blockieren, können zusammen mit antibaktierellen Substanzen bei Infektionskrankheiten eingesetzt werden. Diese Strategie gewinnt zur Zeit an Bedeutung, da Antibiotikaresistenzen immer häufiger auftreten und eine antimikrobielle Behandlung oft nicht mehr ausreicht, um eine Infektion ausreichend zu bekämpfen. Die Inhibierung der Kontaktphasenaktivierung durch Mikroorganismen könnte dazu führen, daß einige Komplikationen, wie Hypotonie und Gerinnungsstörungen, in Patienten mit schwerwiegenden Infektionskrankheiten gemildert werden.

Literatur

1. Pixley RA, Colman RW (1997) The kallikrein-kinin system in sepsis syndrome. In: Farmer SG (ed) Handbook of Immunopharmacology – The Kinin System. Academic Press, New York, pp 173–186
2. Cines DB, Pollak ES, Buck CA et al. (1998) Endothelial cells in physiology and in the pathophysiology of vascular disorders. Blood 91(10):3527–3561
3. Colman RW, Schmaier AH (1997) Contact system: a vascular biology modulator with anticoagulant, profibrinolytic, antiadhesive, and proinflammatory attributes. Blood 90 (10):3819–3843
4. Meijers JC, McMullen BA, Bouma BN (1992) The contact activation proteins: a structure/function overview. Agents Actions Suppl. 38 ((Pt 2)):219–230
5. Reddigari SR, Kuna P, Miragliotta G, Shibayama Y, Nishikawa K, Kaplan AP (1993) Human high molecular weight kininogen binds to human umbilical vein endothelial cells via its heavy and light chains. Blood 8l (5):1306–1311
6. Reddigari SR, Shibayama Y, Brunnee T, Kaplan AP (1993) Human Hageman factor (factor XII) and high molecular weight kininogen compete for the same binding site on human umbilical vein endothelial cells. J Biol Chem 268 (16):11 982–11 987
7. Gustafson EJ, Schmaier AH, Colman RW (1989) High molecular weight kininogen binds to neutrophils. Adv Exp Med Biol 247a:345–348
8. Meloni FJ, Gustafson EJ, Schmaier AH (1992) High molecular weight kininogen binds to platelets by its heavy and light chains and when bound has altered susceptibility to cleavage. Blood 79 (5):1233–1244
9. Meloni FJ, Schmaier AH (1991) Low molecular weight kininogen binds to platelets to modulate thrombin-induced platelet activation. J Biol Chem 266 (11):6786–6794

10. Kaplan AP, Silverberg M (1987) The coagulation-kinin pathway of human plasma. Blood 70 (1): 1–15
11. Bhoola KD, Figueroa CD, Worthy K (1992) Bioregulation of kinins: kallikreins, kininogens, and kininases. Pharmacol Rev 44 (1) 1–80
12. Lottenberg R (1996) Contact activation proteins and the bacterial surface. Trends Microbiol 4 (11): 413–414
13. Mason JW, Kleeberg U, Dolan P, Colman RW (1970) Plasma kallikrein and Hageman factor in Gram-negative bacteremia. Ann Intern Med 73 (4): 545–551
14. Pixley RA, Zellis S, Bankes P et al. (1995) Prognostic value of assessing contact system activation and factor V in systemic inflammatory response syndrome. Crit Care Med 23 (1): 41–51
15. Morrison DC, Roser JF, Henson PM, Cochrane CG (1974) Activation of rat mast cells by low molecular weight stimuli. J Immunol 112 (2): 573–582
16. Minnema MC, Pajkrt D, Wuillemin WA et al. (1998) Activation of clotting factor XI without detectable contact activation in experimental human endotoxemia. Blood 92 (9): 3294–3301
17. Molla A, Yamamoto T, Akaike T, Miyoshi S, Maeda H (1989) Activation of Hageman factor and prekallikrein and generation of kinin by various microbial proteinases. J Biol Chem 264 (18): 10 589–10 594
18. Sakata Y, Akaike T, Suga M, Ijiri S, Ando M, Maeda H (1996) Bradykinin generation triggered by Pseudomonas proteases facilitates invasion of the systemic circulation by *Pseudomonas aeruginosa*. Microbiol Immunol 40 (6): 415–423
19. Maruo K, Akaike, T, Inada Y, Ohkubo I, Ono T, Maeda H (1993) Effect of micorbial and mite proteases on low and high molecular weight kininogens. Generation of kinin and inactivation of thiol protease inhibitory activity. J Biol Chem 268 (24): 17 711–17 715
20. Kadowaki T, Yoneda M, Okamoto K, Maeda K, Yamamoto K (1994) Purification and characterization of a novel arginine-specific cysteine proteinase (argingipain) involved in the pathogenesis of periodontal disease from the culture supernatant of *Porphyromonas gingivalis*. J Biol Chem.269 (33): 21 371–21 378
21. Imamura T, Pike RN, Potempa J, Travis J (1994) Pathogenesis of periodontitis: a major arginine-specific cystein proteinase from Porphyromonas gingivalis induces vascular permeability enhancement through activation of the kinin pathway. J Clin Invest 94 (1): 361–367
22. Scott CF, Whitaker EJ, Hammond BF, Colman RW (1993) Purification and characterization of a potent 70-kDa thiol lysyl-proteinase (Lysgingivain) from *Porphyromonas gingivalis* that cleaves kininogens and fibrinogen. J Biol Chem 268 (11): 7935–7942
23. Herwald H, Collin M, Müller-Esterl W, Björck L (1996) Streptococcal cysteine proteinase releases kinins: a novel virulence mechanism. J Exp Med 184: 665–673
24. Ben Nasr AB, Herwald H, Müller-Esterl W, Björck L (1995) Human kininogens interact with M protein, a bacterial surface protein and virulence determinant. Biochem J 305: 173–180
25. Ben Nasr AB, Olsén A, Sjöbring U, Müller-Esterl W, Björck L (1996) Assembly of human contact phase factors and release of bradykinin at the surface of curle-expressing *Escherichia coli*. Mol Microbiol 20: 927–935
26. Herwald H, Mörgelin M, Olsén A, Rhen M, Dahlbäck B, Müller-Esterl W, Björck L (1998) Activation of the contact phase system on bacterial surfaces – a clue to serious complications in infectious diseases. Nature Medicine 4: 298–302

27. DeLa Cadena RA, Laskin KJ, Pixley RA et al. (1991) Role of kallikrein-kinin system in pathogenesis of bacterial cell wall-induced inflammation. Am J Physiol 260 (2 Pt 1) G213–219
28. Ben Nasr AB, Herwald H, Renné T, Müller-Esterl W, Björck L (1997) Absorption of kininogen from human plasma by *Streptococcus pyogenes* is followed by the release of bradykinin. Biochem J 326:657–660
29. Olsén A, Jonsson A, Normark S (1989) Fibronectin binding mediated by a novel class of surface organelles on *Escherichia coli.* Nature 338 (6217):652–655
30. Collinson SK, Emödy L, Müller KH, Trust TJ, Kay WW (1991) Purification and characterization of thin, aggregative fimbriae from *Salmonella enteritidis.* J Bacteriol 173 (15):4773–4781
31. Olsén A, Wick MJ, Mörgelin M, Björck L (1998) Curli, fibrous surface proteins of *Escherichia coli,* interact with major histocompatibility complex class I molecules. Infect Immun 66:944–949
32. Arnqvist A, Olsén A, Pfeifer J, Russell DG, Normark S (1992) The Crl protein activates cryptic genes for curli formation and fibronetic binding in *Eschericia coli* HB 101. Mol Microbiol 6 (17):2443–2452
33. Olsén A, Arnqvist A, Hammar M, Sukupolvi S, Normark S (1993) The RpoS sigma factor relieves H-NS-mediated transcriptional repression of csgA, the subunit gene of fibronectin-binding curli in *Eschericia coli.* Mol Microbiol 7 (4):523–536
34. Sjöbring U, Pohl G, Olsén A (1994) Plasminogen, absorbed by *Escherichia coli* expressing curli or by *Salmonella enteritidis* expressing thin aggregative fimbriae, can be activated by simultaneously captured tissue-type plasminogen activator (t-PA). Mol Microbiol 14 (3):443–452
35. Imamura T, Potempa J, Pike RN, Travis J (1995) Dependence of vascular permeability enhancement on cysteine proteinases in vesicles of Porphyromonas gingivalis. Infect Immun 63 (5):1999–2003
36. Sakata Y, Akaike T, Khan MM et al. (1996) Activation of bradykinin generating cascade by Vibrio cholerae protease. Immunopharmacology 33 (1–3):377–379
37. Miyoshi N, Miyoshi S, Sugiyama K, Suzuki Y, Furuta H, Shinoda S (1987) Activation of the plasma kallikrein-kinin system by Vibrio vulnificus protease. Infect Immun 55 (8): 1936–1939

Klinik und Intensivtherapie der disseminierten intravasalen Gerinnung

T. Wallner und N. Mayer

Einleitung

Die disseminierte intravasale Gerinnung ist eine potentiell tödlich verlaufende, akzelerierte Aktivierung der Gerinnungskaskade, mit zum Teil noch ungeklärten pathophysiologischen Abläufen. Während klinisch die unstillbare Blutung im Vordergrund steht, ist für die Morbidität die intravasale Bildung von Fibrin mit Thrombosierungen der Mikrozirkulation und dem daraus resultierendem Organversagen entscheidend. Das Phänomen der überschießenden intravasalen Fibrinformation als spezifisches Krankheitscharakteristikum führte zu folgender Neudefinition dieser Hämostasestörung: ***disseminierte intravasale Fibrinformation (DIFF).*** Ein internationaler Konsensus in Bezug auf geeignete labordiagnostische Verfahren und therapeutische Ansätze ist jedoch vorerst nicht in Sicht. Dies liegt zum Teil daran, daß eine Vielzahl von zugrunde liegenden Krankheiten mit unterschiedlichsten klinischen Erscheinungsformen und Laborbefunden eine DIC oder besser DIFF triggern können.

Mit Hilfe neuer molekularer Marker ist es möglich geworden, Gerinnungs- und Fibrinolyseaktivierungen frühzeitig zu erkennen und somit rasch eine adäquate Therapie einzuleiten. Spezifische Testkombinationen eignen sich gut zur Verlaufskontrolle bzw. zum Monitoring des Therapieerfolges. Unerläßlich für die richtige Interpretation der objektiven Laborbefunde und den daraus resultierenden therapeutischen Interventionen, ist jedoch nach wie vor eine große klinische Erfahrung und ärztliche Kompetenz.

Ziel dieser Synopsis ist es, einen klinisch orientierten Leitfaden für den geeigneten diagnostischen und therapeutischen Zugang zu diesem Krankheitsbild zu geben.

Ätiologie und Pathophysiologie

Die disseminierte intravasale Gerinnung ist kein eigenständiges Krankheitsbild, sondern vielmehr ein Syndrom, welches im Zusammenhang mit ganz unterschiedlichen Krankheitsbildern auftreten kann. Im wesentlichen können zwei Entstehungsmechanismen unterschieden werden: das Gewebstrauma und die Schädigung des Gefäßendothels [1]. Traumata unterschiedlicher Genese führen zur Freisetzung von prokoagulatorischem Material (Tissue Factor, TF) in die Zirkulation [2]. Schädigungen des Gefäßendothels mit nachfolgender Aktivierung der Gerinnung sind zumeist die Folge einer Sepsis, die das Einschwemmen von Endotoxin (TNF-α) und ähnlichen Substanzen in die Blutbahn verursacht [3, 4]. Ist das Gerinnungssystem aktiviert, ist der weitere pathophysiologische und klinische Verlauf immer derselbe, unabhängig vom zugrunde liegenden Trigger: Das extrinsische Gerinnungssystem (Faktor VII) wird aktiviert und es kommt durch Interaktion zwischen Gewebsfaktoren (TF) und Faktor VII zur Generierung von Thrombin und nachfolgender Ausbildung von „Fibrin-Clots" [5]. An diesem netzartigen Fibringerinnsel bleiben auch Thrombozyten und Erythrozyten haften und tragen so zur Thrombosierung der Endstrombahn und Endorganschädigung bei [6]. Die gleichzeitig einsetzende überschießende Aktivierung des fibrinolytischen Systems (Plasminaktivierung) führt zwar zur Auflösung der Fibringerinnsel, verursacht aber auch eine Biodegradierung sämtlicher Gerinnungsfaktoren sowie eine Lyse der Thrombozyten und Erythrozyten [7]. Wenn dieser Prozeß ungehindert abläuft und endogene Kompensationsmechanismen versagen, kommt es schließlich zur Blutung. Die disseminierte intravasale Gerinnung (Tabelle 1) ist also initial ein thromboti-

Tabelle 1. Definition der disseminierten intravasalen Gerinnung (Minimalkriterien)

Eine systemisch thrombohämorrhagische Störung in Verbindung mit gut definierten klinischen Situationen und labordiagnostischem Nachweis:
(1) einer Aktivierung des Gerinnungssystems, (2) einer Aktivierung des Fibrinolysesystems, (3) eines Verbrauchs von Inhibitoren, (4) eines Endorganschadens oder -versagens.

(Bick RL (1995) Thromb Haemost 1: 3)

scher Prozeß mit sekundärer, unkontrollierbarer Blutung, die nur auftritt, wenn exzessiv hohe Plasminspiegel zu einer Degradierung von Fibrin, Thrombozyten, Erythrozyten und Gerinnungsfaktoren führen [8].

Klinische Manifestationen

Typischerweise treten als klinisch faßbare Frühsymptome Fieber, Hypotension, Azidose, Hypoxie und Proteinurie auf [9]. Spezifischere Zeichen sind Petechien, akrale Zyanose, Blutungen aus Wunden oder Gefäßpunktionsstellen sowie Blutungen innerer Organe. Vital bedrohlich und von enormer prognostischer Bedeutung sind jedoch nicht die klinisch oft eindrucksvollen Blutungen, sondern vielmehr Mikro- und Makrothrombosierungen, die zu den gefürchteten Organschäden führen. Das Hauptaugenmerk sollte also der Überwachung der Organfunktion gelten. Am häufigsten betroffen sind Herz, Lunge, Niere, Leber und das ZNS [10]. Labordiagnostisch findet man als Hinweis auf eine Organschädigung z. B. erhöhte LDH- oder Kreatininwerte, aber auch erniedrigte PaO_2- und pH-Werte. Verschiedene Kofaktoren beschleunigen die Entwicklung von Mikro- und Makrothrombosierungen: erhöhte Katecholaminspiegel und Vasokonstriktion, Azidose, Glukokortikoide und endogenes ACTH. Die Gabe von Medikamenten sollte daher mit äußerster Vorsicht erfolgen.

Entsprechend dem klinischen und labordiagnostischen Verlauf ist es hilfreich, die disseminierte intravasale Gerinnung in vier verschiedene Phasen einzuteilen, die sich auch als Basis für ein gezieltes Therapiekonzept eignen [11] (Tabelle 2).

Tabelle 2. Klinische Phasen der DIC

Phase I	Aktivierung der Gerinnung
Phase II	Präzipitation und/oder Polymerisation von löslichem Fibrin mit/ohne → Verbrauch von Gerinnungsfaktoren und Inhibitoren → Sekundärer Hyperfibrinolyse
Phase III	Aktivierung und/oder Hemmung der Fibrinolyse Mikrothrombosierung/Thromboembolie und/oder Blutung
Phase IV	Organversagen, unkontrollierbare Blutung

(Müller-Berghaus G et al. (1993) Attempts to define DIC. Excerpta Medica, Amsterdam)

Labordiagnostik

Phase I (Aktivierung der Gerinnung)

Die globalen Gerinnungstests zeigen aufgrund einer Hyperkoagulabilität verkürzte Gerinnungszeiten (Quick↑, aPTT↓). In dieser Phase findet man auch hohe Faktor-Xa- und Thrombinspiegel. Das Akute-Phase-Protein Fibrinogen ist ebenfalls erhöht. Antithrombin beginnt bereits früh zu sinken, während die Thrombin-Antithrombin-Komplexe ansteigen (ATIII↓, TAT↑) (Tabelle 3). ELISA-Assays für die TAT-Bestimmung sind erhältlich. Andere molekulare Marker (s. Tabelle 3), die in Form von Testkits zu Verfügung stehen, sind als Ausdruck erhöhter prokoagulatorischer Aktivität ebenfalls erhöht (s. auch Tabelle 5, Gruppe-1-Tests): Fibrinopeptid A+B (= Maß für die Thrombinaktivität) und das Prothrombinfragment 1+2 (= Maß für die Faktor-Xa-Aktivität). In dieser Phase ist auch bereits eine Thrombozytenreduktion nachweisbar [6, 7, 8]

Tabelle 3. Labordiagnostische Veränderungen entsprechend den vier Phasen der DIC

Phasc	I Hyper- koagulabilität	II Fibrinbildung	III Mikro-/Makro- thrombosierung	IV Organversagen, Blutung
Laborparameter				
Quick	→↑	→	↓	↓↓
aPTT	↓	→	↑	↑↑
TZ	→	→	↑	↑↑
Fibrinogen	↑	→	↓	↓↓
Thrombozyten	→↓	↓	↓↓	↓↓↓
AT III	→↓	↓	↓↓	↓↓↓
TAT	↑	↑↑	↑↑↑	↑↑↑
F1+2	↑	↑↑	↑↑↑	↑↑↑
FM	↑	↑	↑↑	↑↑↑
FDP	→	↑	↑↑	↑↑↑
D-Dimere	→↑	↑	↑↑	↑↑↑

→ unverändert, →↑ unverändert oder erhöht, ↑ erhöht, ↑↑ deutlich erhöht, ↑↑↑ sehr stark erhöht, →↓, unverändert oder erniedrigt, ↓ erniedrigt, ↓↓ deutlich erniedrigt, ↓↓↓ sehr stark erniedrigt, PTT = Partielle Thromboplastinzeit, AT III = Antithrombin III, TAT = Thrombin-Antithrombin-III-Komplex, F1+2 = Prothrombinfragment, FM = Fibrinmonomere, FDP = Fibrinogenspaltprodukte.
(From: Seifried E (1995) Disseminated intravascular coagulation. Hämostaseologie)

Phase II (Fibrinbildung und reaktive Aktivierung der Fibrinolyse)

Die Polymerisation der Fibrinmonomere führt zur Bildung von löslichem Fibrin und Fibringerinnsel. Gleichzeitig setzt die Hyperfibrinolyse ein. Dies führt häufig zu einer Normalisierung der globalen Gerinnungstests, während AT-III-Spiegel und Thrombozytenzahlen weiter sinken (s. Tabelle 3). Die sehr sensitiven Molekularmarker der Hyperfibrinolyse werden positiv (s. Tabelle 5): z. B. Fibrinogen-Spaltprodukte (FDP), die durch die Einwirkung von Plasmin auf Fibrinogen entstehen. Fibrinogen-Spaltprodukte können sich mit Fibrinmonomeren (FM) zu FDP-FM-Komplexen verbinden, genannt ***lösliches Fibrin*** [12]. Diese Komplexe bilden die Basis für den Protamin-Sulfat-Test [13].

Die Zuverlässigkeit der globalen Gerinnungstests in der Phase I und II beträgt nur etwa 50% und ist daher für die Frühdiagnose der DIC von untergeordneter Bedeutung [6–8]! Die verläßlichsten Tests für die Frühdiagnose sind in Tabelle 4 aufgelistet.

Phase III (Mikrothrombosierung und Blutung)

Mikrothrombosierung, Verbrauch bzw. proteolytische Degradierung von Gerinnungsfaktoren und anhaltende Hyperfibrinolyse charakterisieren die dritte Phase. Die globalen Gerinnungstests bestätigen die inzwischen klinisch manifesten Blutungen (Quick ↓↓, aPTT ↑↑, TZ ↓↓), Thrombozytenzahlen und AT-III-Spiegel sind drastisch erniedrigt (s. Tabelle 3). Molekulare Fibrinolysemarker sind stark erhöht (Tabelle 5), vor allem Fibrinogen-Spaltprodukte und D-Dimere [15].

Phase IV (Multiorganversagen und exzessive Blutung)

Alle Molekularmarker steigen weiter an, exzessive Blutungen und die Auswirkungen der Organschäden prägen das dramatische Bild in diesem Stadium.

Tabelle 4. Wichtige labordiagnostische Bestimmungen für die DIC

D-Dimer[a]	FDP[a]	Thrombozytenzahl	Fibrinogen
Antithrombin[a]	Fibrinopeptid A[a]	Protamintest	Prothrombinzeit
F. 1+2[a]	Plättchenfaktor 4[a]	Thrombinzeit	aPTT

[a] Die verläßlichsten Teste. (Bick RL (1996) Semin Thromb Hemostas 22/1)

Tabelle 5. Labordiagnostische Kriterien[a]

Diese Tests sind zum Nachweis einer prokoagulatorischen Aktivität geeignet (Gruppe-1-Tests):

- erhöhtes Prothrombinfragment 1+2
- erhöhtes Fibrinopeptid A
- erhöhtes Fibrinopeptid B
- erhöhte Thrombin-Antithrombin-Komplexe (TAT)
- erhöhte D-Dimere[b]

Diese Tests sind zum Nachweis einer Fibrinolyseaktivierung geeignet (Gruppe-2-Tests):

- erhöhte D-Dimere
- erhöhte FDP
- erhöhte Plasminspiegel
- erhöhte Plasmin-Antiplasmin-Komplexe (PAP)

Diese Tests sind zum Nachweis des Inhibitorenverbrauches geeignet (Gruppe-3- Tests):

- erniedrigtes AT III
- erniedrigtes alpha-2-Antiplasmin
- erniedrigter Heparin-Kofaktor II
- erniedrigte Protein C- oder S-Spiegel
- erhöhte TAT-Komplexe
- erhöhte PAP-Komplexe

Diese Tests sind zum Nachweis eines Organschadens geeignet (Gruppe-4-Tests):

- erhöhtes LDH
- erhöhtes Kreatinin
- erniedrigter pH-Wert
- vermindertes PaO_2

[a] Nur ein pathologischer Befund ist notwendig in Gruppe 1, 2 und 3, während zumindest zwei pathologische Befunde in Gruppe 4 notwendig sind, um eine DIC verläßlich labordiagnostisch bestätigen zu können.

[b] Der D-Dimer-Test ist in diesem Zusammenhang nur verläßlich, wenn der „Connect-Assay“ und monoklonale Antikörper verwendet werden. (Bick RL (1996) Semin Thromb Hemostas 22/1)

Hochgradige Azidose, Hypoxie als Ausdruck der Hämolyse sowie Thrombozytenzahlen von weniger als 2000/µl sind labordiagnostische Korrelate.

Zusammenfassend kann man sagen, daß zur objektiven Diagnose der DIC, in Entsprechung der vier Phasen, die in Tabelle 5 zusammengestellten Test-Kombinationen benötigt werden:

- Prokoagulatorische Aktivierung (Gruppe-1-Tests),
- Aktivierung der Fibrinolyse (Gruppe-2-Tests),
- Verbrauch der Inhibitoren (Gruppe-3-Tests),
- Organschädigung (Gruppe-4-Tests).

Therapie der DIC

Das vorrangige therapeutische Ziel ist die Elimination der auslösenden Grunderkrankung, die für die Entwicklung der hämostaseologischen Entgleisung verantwortlich gemacht wird [16]. Die primäre Behandlung und Korrektur pathologischer Gerinnungsparameter erweist sich oft als frustran, solange nicht der Trigger eliminiert wurde. Es konnte beispielsweise gezeigt werden, daß eine Uterusextirpation bei geburtshilflichen Komplikationen mit DIC, zu einem sofortigem Sistieren des intravasalen Thrombosierungsprozesses führt [17]. Erst nach erfolgreicher Behandlung des auslösenden Triggers führt die Substitution der im Anschluß beschriebenen Hämostasetherapeutika zur Normalisierung der Gerinnungsstörung.

Phase I

Da die Hyperkoagulabilität der dominierende Prozeß in dieser Phase ist, sind Antikoagulantien und Gerinnungsinhibitoren indiziert. Heparin in niedriger Dosierung von ca. 150–200 I.E./kg KG/Tag oder 10000–15000 I.E./Tag wird erfolgreich eingesetzt [18]. Heparin kann sowohl intravenös als auch subkutan gegeben werden. Für die subkutane Gabe wird eine Dosis von 80–100 I.E./kg KG alle 4–6 Stunden empfohlen [19]. Die subkutane Low-dose-Heparintherapie hat mehrere Vorteile: Sie birgt kaum die Gefahr einer Blutungsneigung, höhere Dosen können jederzeit verabreicht werden und die subkutane Applikation scheint genauso effektiv zu sein wie hohe intravenöse Dosen. Die Effizienz dieser Therapie zeigt sich an einer Zunahme der AT-III- und Fibrinogenspiegel sowie einer Abnahme der FDP-Konzentrationen [14]. Im allgemeinen wird jedoch diese frühe Phase der prokoagulatorischen Aktivität in Ermangelung klinischer Auffälligkeiten nicht rechtzeitig erkannt.

Phase II

Die begonnene Heparintherapie sollte weiter geführt werden (Tabelle 6). Als das Therapeutikum der ersten Wahl für die moderate und fulminante DIC gilt Antithrombin III, das in dieser Phase zusätzlich gegeben werden sollte [20]. Es gilt folgende Dosierungsrichtlinie:

$$(\text{angestrebte} - \text{aktuelle AT-III-Konzentration in \%}) \times \text{kg KG} = \text{I.E. AT III}$$

Der angestrebte Wert sollte etwa 80–100% (besser 125%) betragen, und die Substitution sollte alle 8 Stunden (2000–4000 I.E./24 h) erfolgen [14]. Grundsätzlich kommen auch andere Antikoagulantien in Betracht: rekombinante Hirudine [21] Defibrotide [22], Gabexate [23], humanes lösliches Thrombomodulin, D-TFPI (ein Faktor-VIIa-Hemmer) oder DX-9065a (ein Faktor-Xa-Hemmer). Ein anderes experimentelles und kostspieliges Agens ist das Protein-C-Konzentrat, welches bei der Therapie der gramnegativen Sepsis in naher Zukunft zum Einsatz kommen soll. Alle diese Substanzen sind jedoch noch nicht klinisch erprobt.

Phase III

Die in diesem Stadium klinisch apparenten Blutungen sind durch eine Depletion von Gerinnungsfaktoren sowie durch Thrombozytopenie und Hyperfibrinolyse bedingt.

Tabelle 6. Sequentielle Therapie der DIC entsprechend der vier Phasen

Phase	I	II	III	IV
Heparin	+	+	(+)	
FFP		+	+	+
AT III		+	+	+
PPSB			(+)	+
Fibrinogen				(+)[a]
F XIII				(+)
Thrombozyten			(+)	+
Antifibrinolytika				+[a]
Erythrozytenkonzentrate		(+)	(+)	+

[a] Ultima ratio. (Seifried E (1995) Hämostaseologie 15/2:57–64)

Trotzdem sollte die Substitution von Gerinnungsfaktoren und diverser anderer Komponenten auch im Vollbild der DIC mit äußerster Vorsicht erfolgen. Wenn Vollblut, FFP oder Kryopräzipitate einem Patienten mit manifester DIC gegeben werden, kommt es – bedingt durch die Einwirkung der enorm hohen Plasminkonzentrationen – zu einer sofortigen Biodegradierung sämtlicher Gerinnungsfaktoren. Das ist zwar nicht gefährlich, aber keinesfalls sinnvoll. Von größerer Bedeutung ist aber, daß diese Produkte Fibrinogen enthalten und somit zur Bildung noch höherer FDP-Konzentrationen beitragen. Diese Spaltprodukte (FDP) verbinden sich wiederum mit Fibrinmonomer-Polymerisaten zu Fibrinthromben und führen dadurch zur weiteren mikro- und makrovaskulären Thrombosierung und Thrombozytenzerstörung [14]. Solange also die AT-III-Konzentrationen nicht im Normalbereich sind (>80%), müssen alle verabreichten Derivate frei von Fibrinogen sein [6, 7, 8]. Als sichere Produkte in der Therapie der unkontrollierten DIC mit niedrigen AT-III-Spiegel gelten Erythrozytenkonzentrate, Thrombozytenkonzentrate und ungerinnbare proteinhaltige Plasmaexpander, wie Plasmaproteinfraktionen (PPF), Humanalbumin und Hydroxyäthylstärke [25]. Bei normalen AT-III-Werten (100–125%) können gefahrlos sämtliche Derivate und Produkte gegeben werden: FFP zur prokoagulatorischen Aktivierung, AT III als wichtigsten Gerinnungshemmer und Prothrombinkomplexe (PPSB), falls die Substitution mit FFP nicht ausreicht (Tabelle 7). Die Gabe von Prothrombinkomplexen wird allerdings kontrovers diskutiert und von manchen Autoren auch als „Öl ins Feuer gießen" angesehen [25]. Erythrozyten- und Thrombozytenkonzentrate werden je nach Laborbefund ersetzt, die Heparintherapie sollte je nach klinischer Situation entweder gestoppt oder auf etwa 35–75 I.E./kg KG/Tag reduziert werden [11].

Phase IV

Führen diese sequentiellen therapeutischen Schritte dennoch nicht zum Sistieren der Thrombose- und Blutungsneigung, empfiehlt sich folgendes Vorgehen. FFP, AT III und PPSB werden weiter substituiert. Thrombozytenkonzentrate müssen bei einer Thrombopenie von 10 000–20 000/μl verabreicht werden, wobei dies aufgrund der verkürzten Lebensdauer der Thrombozyten in immer kürzeren Intervallen erforderlich wird. Fibrinogenkonzentrate sind bei Werten um 50 mg/dl indiziert [6–8]. Faktor-XIII-Konzentrate, notwendig zur Quervernetzung von Fibrinmonomeren, können im Einzelfall hilfreich sein, wenn die Konzentration auf unter 30% abfällt [11]. Als nächster Schritt ist die Hemmung

Tabelle 7. Therapie der DIC; Dosierungen

Heparin	Phase I 150–200 I.E.i.v./kg/Tag oder 10 000–15 000 I.E./Tag Phase III 35–70 I.E./kg/Tag oder 2500–5000 I.E./Tag
Fresh frozen plasma (FFP)	4–10 I.E. i.v./Tag → AT III >80% (80–125%)
AT III	2000 I.E. i.v. Bolus → AT III >80% (80–125%) 2000–4000 I.E. i.v./Tag
PPSB	2000–4000 I.E. i.v./Tag → PT >30%
Fibrinogen	2–4g i.v.Bolus → Fibrinogen >50 mg/dl
FXIII	20–40 I.E. i.v./Tag → F XIII >30%
Thrombozyten	6–10 Konzentrate/Tag → Thrombozyten >10 000/Bl
Antifibrinolytika:	
Aprotinin	500 000 I.E. i.v. Bolus 50 000–200 000 I.E. i.v./Stunde
Tranexamsäure	0,5–1g i.v. als Infusion 0,125–0,5g i.v./Stunde
Erykonzentrate	2–4 Konzentrate/tag

Die empfohlenen Dosen sollten individuell und den klinisch-labordiagnostischen Befunden angepaßt werden. (Seifried E (1995) Hämostaseologie 15/2:57–64)

der sekundären Hyperfibrinolyse durch Antifibrinolytika in Betracht zu ziehen. Dies ist allerdings nur in etwa 3% der Fälle erforderlich und sollte keinesfalls routinemäßig durchgeführt werden, weil dadurch möglicherweise der Thrombosierung Vorschub geleistet wird. Es wurden tödliche Lungenembolien nach Gabe von Antifibrinolytika in Fallberichten publiziert [27]. Lege artis darf eine antifibrinolytische Therapie nur eingeleitet werden, wenn ein hoher Plasminspiegel, weitgehender Fibrinogenverlust oder eine starke Verminderung von funktionellem Plasminogen und α2-PI dokumentiert ist. Dies ist beispielsweise durch Bestimmung der PAP-Komplexe möglich. Als Therapeutika stehen Epsilon-Aminocapronsäure, Tranexamsäure oder Aprotinin zu Verfügung. Epsilon-Aminocapronsäure wird zunächst in einer Dosierung von 5–10 g langsam intravenös verabreicht, danach Repetitionsdosen von 2–4 g/h über 24 Stunden oder bis zum Sistieren der Blutungen. Alternativ können 500 000 I.E. Aprotinin als Bolus, oder 50 000–200 000 I.E./Tag gegeben werden. Da Aprotinin auch eine antikoagulatorische Wirkung hat, ist die Gefahr der Bildung disseminierter Thrombosen geringer.

Zusammenfassung

Durch den Einsatz neuer Molekularmarker ist es möglich, die DIC schon in ihrer Entstehungsphase zu diagnostizieren. Die Auswahl geeigneter Testkombinationen und die richtige Interpretation der hoch spezifischen Laboranalysen ermöglichen ein ganz gezieltes therapeutisches Eingreifen. Die Eliminierung der Grundkrankheit bleibt allerdings die conditio sine qua non für eine erfolgreiche Behandlung der hämostaseologischen Entgleisung. Hyperkoagulabilität und Hyperfibrinolyse müssen möglichst effizient kompensiert werden, um irreversible Organschäden zu vermeiden. Die antifibrinolytische Therapie ist als ultima ratio anzusehen und sollte nur im äußerstem Notfall und nach labordiagnostischem Beweis für das Vorliegen einer Hyperfibrinolyse angewandt werden. Trotz aller diagnostischer und therapeutischer Fortschritte, die in den letzten Jahren gemacht wurden, bleibt die Behandlung dieses lebensbedrohlichen Syndroms eine große Herausforderung.

Literatur

1. Kirchmaier CM (1995) Etiology and pathophysiology of disseminated intravascular coagulation. Hämostaseologie 15:69–78
2. Hardaway RM (1980) Mechanism of traumatic shock. Surg Gynecol Obstet 151:65–69
3. Colman RW (1994) Disseminated intravascular coagulation due to sepsis. Semin Hematol 31/2 (Suppl 1):10–17
4. Mammen EF (1993) Inhibitor substitution in septicemia. Prospectives for the future. Intensive Care Med 19 (Suppl 1):29–34
5. Bell WR (1994) The pathophysiology of disseminated intravascular coagulation. Semin Hematol 31:19–25
6. Bick RL (1988) Disseminated intravascular coagulation and related syndromes: A clinical review. Semin Thromb Hemostas 14:299
7. Bick RL, Baker WF (1992) Disseminated intravascular coagulation. Hematol Pathol 6:1
8. Bick RL (1992) Disseminated intravascular coagulation. In: Bick RL (ed) Disorders of thrombosis and hemostasis. Clinical and laboratory practice. ASCP Press, Chicago, p 137
9. Baker WF (1989) Clinical aspects of disseminated intravascular coagulation: A clinician's point of view. Thromb Hemostas 15:1
10. Müller-Berghaus G (1977) Pathophysiology of generalized intravascular coagulation. Semin Thromb Hemostas 3:209
11. Seifried E (1995) Disseminierte intravasale Gerinnung. Diagnostik und Therapie in der klinischen Praxis. Hämostaseologie 15/2:57–64
12. Bang NU, Chang M (1974) Soluble fibrin complexes. Semin Thromb Hemostas 1:91
13. Gurewich V, Lipinsky B, Lipinska I (1973) A comparative study of precipitation paracoagulation by protamine sulfate and ethanol gelation test. Thromb Res 539

14. Bick RL (1996) Disseminated intravascular coagulation: Objective clinical and laboratory diagnosis, treatment, and assessment of therapeutic response. Semin Thromb Hemostas 22/1:69–88
15. Myers AR, Bloch KJ, Coleman RW (1970) A comparative study of four methods for detecting fibrinogen degradation products in patients with various diseases. N Engl J Med 283:633
16. Feinstein DI (1988) Treatment of disseminated intravascular coagulation. Semin Thromb Hemostas 14:351
17. Beller FK, Uszynski M (1974) Disseminated intravascular coagulation in pregnancy. Clin Obstet Gynecol 27:250–278
18. Du Toit HJ, Coetzee AR, Chalton DO (1991) Heparin treatment in thrombin induced disseminated intravascular coagulation in the baboon. Crit Care Med
19. Bentley BG, Kakkar VV et al. (1980) An objective study of alternative methods of heparin administration. Thromb Res 18:177
20. Bick RL, Fekete LF (1976) Treatment of disseminated intravascular coagulation with antithrombin III. Trans Am Soc Hematol:167
21. Talbot M (1989) Biology of recombinant hirudin (CGP 39393): A new prospect in the treatment of thrombosis. Semin Thromb Hemostas 15:293
22. Niada R, Prota R et al. (1989) Thrombolytic activity of defibrotide against old venous thrombi. Semin Thromb Hemostas 15:474
23. Umeki S, Adachi M et al. (1988) Gabexate as a therapy of disseminated intravascular coagulation. Arch Intern Med 148:1409
24. Yamazaki M, Asakura H, Aoshima K et al. (1994) Effects of DX-9065-a, an orally active, newly synthesized and specific inhibitor of factor Xa, against experimental disseminated intravascular coagulation in rats. Thromb Hemostas 72:393–396
25. Bick RL, Schmalhorst WR, Fekete LF (1976) Disseminated intravascular coagulation and blood component therapy. Transfusion 16:361
26. Bick RL (1992) Disseminated intravascular coagulation. Hematol Oncol Clin North Am 6:1259
27. Staudinger T, Locker GJ, Frass M (1996) Management of acquired coagulation disorders in emergency and intensive care medicine. Semin Thromb Hemostas 22/1:93–103

CHAPTER 5

The Inflammatory Effect of Coagulation and the Antiinflammatory Effect of Anticoagulation in Sepsis and Shock

I. Pneumatikos and A. B. J. Groeneveld

Introduction

It is estimated from circulating levels of coagulation and fibrinolysis activators (and inhibitors) and breakdown products that many, but not all, patients with sepsis and allied conditions show evidence of diffuse intravascular coagulation (DIC) that may contribute, by thrombin generation, widespread microvascular fibrin deposits and platelet aggregates, to development of multiple organ damage and ultimate demise [1, 2]. The DIC may involve activation of coagulation and activation and subsequent inhibition of fibrinolysis, which are, in part, regulated differently. Activation of inflammatory cascades, including release of cytokines such as tumor necrosis factor (TNF-α), may lead to harmful activation of the coagulation cascade via tissue factor synthesis, while the contact system and factor XII activation may contribute to hypotension and inhibition of activated fibrinolysis.

The circulating levels of endogenous anticoagulants such as proteins S and C and antithrombin III (ATIII) are decreased following consumption or suppression, while circulating tissue factor pathway inhibitor (TFPI) and the protein C cofactor thrombomodulin may be increased following release by endothelium damaged by activated neutrophils, and these changes may be predictive for major complications and death from sepsis [2]. Neutrophil-derived proteolytic enzymes may also inactivate anticoagulants, such as TFPI, ATIII, and heparin, and heparin may enhance inactivation of ATIII by elastase [3]. Abnormalities may be even more severe in some animal models of sepsis. For a full description of the sepsis and inflammation-induced activation of coagulation and (inhibition of) activated fibrinolysis, the reader is referred to other texts [2]. Inflammatory responses, on the other hand, could also have some anticoagulant effects via the liberation of nitric oxide (NO), an inhibitor of platelet and neutrophil aggregation and adhesion, and of fibrinolysis inhibition [4]. NO may also inhibit tissue factor synthesis in monocytes [5]. In fact, the administration of NO synthase blockers in animal models of endotoxin shock and increased vessel wall NO production may result in widespread intravascular thrombosis [6].

In this review, we will collectively describe the evidence that coagulation activates inflammation and that anticoagulant therapy, in conditions with DIC such as sepsis and shock, may attenuate inflammatory responses. In fact, DIC could aggravate inflammatory responses and thereby contribute to their potentially harmful effect. Hence, strategies have been developed, mainly in experimental studies, that aim to limit (evidence of) DIC and thereby the inflammatory responses, development of multiple organ dysfunction, and ultimate death by anticoagulant measures. Multicenter studies are underway that explore the potential benefit of various anticoagulants proven to be efficacious in animals and in human sepsis and allied conditions.

Coagulation Induces an Inflammatory Response

By acting on the neutrophil and the endothelium and by increasing permeability and adhesiveness, thrombin generation during activation of coagulation following inflammation may amplify the inflammatory response at the level of neutrophil endothelial interactions, and thereby contribute to organ damage. For instance, thrombin infusion may evoke a pulmonary microvascular injury. Ostrovsky et al. [7] demonstrated in mesenteric ischemic/reperfusion in cats that thrombin plays an important role in leukocyte rolling and adhesion during reperfusion. Drake et al. [8] found that thrombin synergistically enhanced the neutrophil transendothelial migration induced by interleukin (IL)-1α and TNF-α through human umbilical vein endothelial cells and in rabbit skin.

Thrombin may generate a cytokine response. In whole blood, Johnson et al. [9] found that whole blood coagulation in vitro evoked cytokine release, particularly of IL-8, rather than of TNF-α and IL-1β, and partially mediated by thrombin. The combination of coagulation plus endotoxin resulted in significantly greater IL-8 production. The addition of TFPI or other anticoagulants to the whole blood abrogated IL-8 production induced by coagulation or coagulation plus endotoxin. This study shows the cross-talk between coagulation and cytokines cascades in whole blood and indentifies IL-8 as the key inflammatory participant. Thrombin may, finally, help to cleave endothelium-derived IL-8 into a smaller but more active form [10]. Indeed, IL-8 may be a principal cytokine released during coagulation activation in the course of sepsis and lung injury in patients [1]. Others [11], however, found IL-1β expression in coagulated whole blood samples from healthy volunteers. Conversely, anticoagulation of whole blood with EDTA may limit endotoxin-induced monocyte, neutrophil, and platelet activation responses and tissue factor, cytokine, and lactoferrin releases, as compared to anticoagulation with other substances including heparin [12].

Fibrin has been found to enhance the expression of IL-1β by human monocytes [13]. Fibrin matrices may suppress the expression of endogenous cytokine competitors such as IL-1 receptor antagonist, thus enhancing proinflammatory effects. Fibrin may also activate IL-8 expression and thereby induce neutrophil chemotaxis in endothelial cells in vitro [14]. These findings add fibrin to the list of extracellular matrix components capable of modulating the inflammatory response to injury. Nevertheless, others have suggested that fibrinogen inhibits rather than enhances neutrophil chemotactic activity in response to stimulants such as IL-8 [15]. Finally, Robson et al. [16] observed that D-dimer, a terminal degradation product of fibrin, induced synthesis and release of IL-1β, IL-6, and plasminogen activator inhibitor by human monocytes.

Activated Platelets

Platelet activation may synergize with leukocyte activation in tissue damage during sepsis [17–19]. This may partly relate to increased platelet–neutrophil/monocyte and leukocyte–endothelium interactions [20]. For instance, some authors [17, 21] have shown that (thrombin-) stimulated platelets activate neutrophils and monocytes in human cell suspensions and whole blood in a contact-dependent manner to secrete neutrophil products and cytokines such as IL-8 but not tissue factor, respectively. Fibrinogen and P selectin exposure on the platelet surface seems to be necessary for this interaction and activation, but other neutrophil agonists may also play a role [17, 21, 22]. Indeed, Hawrylowicz et al. [23] showed that suspensions of washed human platelets express IL-1 activity on the membrane after activation with thrombin and others agents. In fact, other authors [24] found that platelets activated in vitro via IL-1 on their membranes induce endothelial secretion of IL-8 and adhesion molecules. Platelet blockade by aspirin may prevent this effect.

Anticoagulation Inhibits the Inflammatory Response

The natural circulating anticoagulants, such as proteins C and S and ATIII, inhibit activation of fibrin generation. Tissue factor pathway inhibitors or antibodies have been developed to block the first step in the coagulation activation cascade during sepsis. Conversely, the naturally circulating fibrinolysis activators such as tissue plasminogen activator and urokinase activate the conversion of plasminogen to plasmin, thereby promoting fibrinolysis. Exogenously administered heparin may mainly act as an ATIII activator, while low-molecular-weight heparanoids mainly act as factor X inhibitors. These anticoagulant/fibrinolytic factors may have antiinflammatory effects, via leukocytes and endothelium, that may be relevant in the treatment of inflammatory disorders accompanied by widespread intravasular coagulation, organ dysfunction, and death. In fact, administration of the inactive derivate of factor Xa (DEGR-Xa), a selective inhibitor of thrombin generation, or heparin prevented the coagulopathic response but did not prevent the cytokine (TNF-α) response, organ damage, shock and death in baboons made septic by *Escherichia coli* infusion, or in rats with endotoxin infusion [25–27]. This may indicate that the protective effects of the anticoagulants discussed below can be partially attributed to other effects than anticoagulant ones.

Tissue Factor Pathway Inhibitor/Antibodies

The TFPI is a naturally occurring protein synthesized by endothelial cells, among others. It may inhibit activated factor Xa directly and factor VIIa/tissue factor activity by forming a quartenary Xa/TFPI/Va complex. It may prevent a cytokine response to coagulation of whole blood in vitro [9].

In an early study, Taylor and associates observed that pretreatment with a tissue-factor-blocking antibody prevented lethal shock in *E. coli*-infected baboons [28]. A similar survival benefit was shown in mice injected with endotoxin, but the rise in circulating TNF-α was not attenuated [29]. In endotoxin-challenged chimpanzees also, tissue factor or factor VII/VIIa antibody pretreatment attenuated coagulation but not the cytokine response [30]. In a study by Creasey et al. [31] of lethal *E. coli*-induced shock in baboons, early posttreatment of recombinant TFPI resulted in permanent survivors and significant attenuations of the coagulation response and various measures of organ dysfunction. Moreover, TFPI-treated, *E. coli*-infected baboons had significantly lower IL-6 plasma levels than controls but TNF-α levels were similarly elevated in both groups. Similar results were obtained with a different recombinant preparation of TFPI [32]. Finally, recombinant TFPI may bind endotoxin, thereby attenuating cellular response to the latter [33]. The data thus suggest that TFPI is able to inhibit not only the intravascular coagulation but also the inflammatory response in sepsis and DIC. TFPI is currently being evaluated in clinical trials.

Protein C

Thrombomodulin is an endothelial cell-membrane glycoprotein that contributes to regulation of the coagulation system by binding thrombin and accelerating the thrombin-catalyzed activation of protein C. Activated protein C (aPC) proteolytically inactivates the coagulation cofactors Va and VIIIa and promotes fibrinolysis by complex formation with plasminogen activator inhibitor.

Taylor et al. [34] demonstrated that infusion of aPC prevents the coagulopathic response and lethal effects of *E. coli*-induced shock in baboons. They also found that blocking protein C activation in vivo led to a more severe response, prevented by coinfusion of aPC. In a rat study by Murakami et al. [27], administration of aPC prevented the endotoxin-induced increase in pulmonary vascular permeability by reducing pulmonary accumulation of leukocytes. Neither ATIII plus heparin nor DEGR-Xa were effective, while they attenuated coagulation. Finally, recombinant thrombomodulin may have a similar action in this model [26]. Thrombomodulin was also effective in endotoxin-induced DIC in rats [35].

The precise (antiinflammatory?) mechanism of action of aPC has not been fully elucidated. Grey et al. demonstrated that aPC, even though preventing downregulation of endotoxin receptor expression, diminished TNF-α release by endotoxin-activated monocytes in vitro [36, 37]. Endotoxin may also activate thrombomodulin release by human monocytes [36], so that extravascular macrophages may promote local production of aPC upon stimulation. In fact, aPC may diminish TNF-α release and promote survival in endotoxin shock in rodents [36]. The combination of ATIII and protein C posttreatment in endotoxic shock in pigs attenuated the TNF-α but not the IL-6 increase in plasma, while ameliorating hypotension [38].

These observations provided a rationale for the use of protein C in the treatment of septic shock associated with DIC. A beneficial effect of protein C in humans with meningococcal sepsis and DIC has been suggested by several case reports [39, 40]. Infusion of protein C has led to cessation of the progress of the skin lesions and a rapid improvement in the patients' condition.

Antithrombin III

ATIII is an endogenous regulator of blood coagulation. It inhibits thrombin and factors IXa, Xa, and XIa by forming irreversible complexes. The inhibitory reaction is accelerated by endothelial surface proteoglycanes or by exogenously administered heparin.

Until recently, the proposed mode of action of ATIII in patients with sepsis was mainly restricted to the anticoagulant activity of the drug. In 1984 Triantafylopoulos noted that ATIII pretreatment significantly increased the survival of endotoxin-infused rabbits without improving coagulopathy [41]. In fact, the evidence is accumulating that there is an additional antiinflammatory action of ATIII apart from its anticoagulant properties. Taylor et al. have demonstrated that preinfusion of ATIII reduced the coagulopathy and cell injury responses and prevented death in baboons given a lethal dose of live *E. coli*, while blocking coagulation with DEGR-Xa alone had no effect on survival [25, 42]. This indicates that the lifesaving effect of ATIII in this animal model may not have been caused by blocking fibrin formation. Kessler et al. [43] found that ATIII decreased evidence of DIC and mortality of guinea pigs following *Staphylococcus aureus* infusion. Low-molecular-weight heparin coinfusion partially abrogated the beneficial response of ATII because of binding to ATIII. The combination of ATIII and protein C posttreatment in endotoxic shock in pigs attenuated the TNF-α but not the IL-6 increase in plasma, while ameliorating hypotension [38].

The potential antiinflammatory action of ATIII may be partly attributed to the release of prostacyclin from endothelial cells after the interaction of ATIII with heparin-like glycosaminoglycanes (GAGs) on the endothelial cell surface, which may accelerate thrombin binding [44–46]. This may be evidenced by a rise in the circulating levels of prostglandin breakdown products [45–47]. The activities of prostacyclin include vasodilation, inhibition of platelet activation, inhibition of leukocyte activation by reducing TNF-α and oxygen radical production, and inhibition of neutrophil adhesion to the endothelial cells.

In rats given intravenous endotoxin, Uchiba et al. demonstrated that intravenous ATIII inhibited pulmonary neutrophil accumulation and increased permeability, concomitantly with a rise in prostaglandin breakdown products in the blood [46, 47]. This was not inhibited by DEGR-Xa, selectively inhibiting thrombin generation, nor by combined use of heparin and ATIII [27]. The latter was likely the result of heparin binding to ATIII and preventing ATIII from interacting with heparin-like GAGs on the endothelial cell surface [27, 45, 46]. The therapeutic effects of ATIII on pulmonary vascular injury in rats given endotoxin were not observed after pretreatment with indomethacin to prevent the synthesis of prostacyclin from endothelial cells [46]. Although high-dose ATIII prevented endotoxin-induced pulmonary vascular injury and coagulation abnormalities in rats, the lower dose prevented coagulopathy but not pulmonary vascular injury [47]. These observations suggest that the ATIII dose required to prevent endothelial cell injury is higher than that needed to inhibit coagulation abnormalities in animal models of sepsis [48].

The dual mechanism of action of ATIII suggested above, which is anticoagulant and antiinflammatory, has prompted studies on possible beneficial effects of the drug, which should be administered in large doses to obtain supranormal circulating ATIII levels, in patients with severe sepsis. Investigators [49, 50] observed that plasma levels of cytokines IL-6 and IL-8, adhesion molecules and C1 reactive protein were lower in sepsis (and polytrauma) patients who received ATIII treatment than in sepsis patients who did not receive such treatment. A recent metanalysis of three double-blind placebo-controlled phase II trials on ATIII in patients with severe sepsis resulted in a 23% reduction in 30-day all-cause mortality [51]. Other studies may confirm this [52]. In the ongoing phase III trial the beneficial role of ATIII in severe sepsis should be proven, before routine clinical use can be recommended.

Other Models

Recently, Ostrovsky et al. [7] demonstrated in mesenteric ischemia/reperfusion (I/R) in cats that pre- and posttreatment with ATIII reduced neutrophil rolling and adhesion to preischemic levels during reperfusion. Vascular hyperpermeability was also reduced by ATIII. Harada et al. [53] showed that ATIII, given before reperfusion, can reduce I/R-induced injury of rat liver by increasing hepatic blood flow and inhibiting leukocyte activation, possibly mediated via increased prostacyclin generation, since indomethacin abrogated the effect of ATIII. Neither DEGR-XA nor modified, and thus inactive, ATIII had such an effect.

Bleeker et al. [54] investigated the effect of ATIII in a lethal pancreatitis model induced by taurocholate in rats. The compound, given either prophylactically or therapeutically, appeared to improve the otherwise 85% mortality rate at 30 h after induction. In a similar model of pancreatitis, Yamachuchi et al. [55] demonstrated that neither pre- nor posttreatment with C1 esterase inhibitor or ATIII monotherapy could increase survival. The combination (pre or post) therapy, however, improved survival.

Heparin and Heparin-like Substances

Apart from its anticoagulant properties, heparin may have antiinflammatory actions. Heparin anticoagulation may suppress endotoxin-induced TNF-α, IL-1β, IL-6, tissue factor and plasminogen activator inhibitor expression and release in isolated monocytes [56, 57]. Low-molecular-weight heparin may be less active in this respect [58].

Nevertheless, anticoagulation of whole blood with heparin may not limit endotoxin-induced monocyte, neutrophil, and platelet activation responses, as compared to anticoagulation with EDTA [12]. In fact, heparin may activate neutrophil adhesion molecules and IL-8, but not at high doses, in vitro [59]. In the study by Miller et al. [60], heparin has been found to downregulate the expression of adhesion molecules in human endothelial cells in vitro. Nevertheless, heparin may enhance neutrophilic chemotactic responses to IL-8 but may inhibit elastase release in vitro [61]. Low-molecular-weight heparins may also bind to adhesion molecules and inhibit neutrophil adhesiveness and transmigration in inflammation in vivo [57]. Finally, Lantz et al. [62] suggested that heparin and heparin-like molecules of the extracellular matrix can retain TNF-α in physical proximity with target cells in the interstitium. In this way, heparin-like molecules may restrict the actions of TNF-α and protect against systemic harmful manifestations. Taken together, heparin may have a complex role in the transendothelial trafficking and activation of leukocytes.

Heparin pretreatment or perfusion may prevent endotoxin-induced liver injury in rats, partly via thrombin inhibition [63]. In the rats studied by Morrison et al. [64] after cecal ligation and puncture, heparin and a novel nonanticoagulant heparin (GM 1892) prevented decreased acetylcholine-induced vascular relaxation during the hyperdynamic stage of sepsis. In *Staphylococcus aureus*-infused guinea pigs, infusion of low-molecular-weight heparin hardly improved morbidity and mortality [43]. In contrast, low-molecular weight heparin pretreatment prevented TNF-α release and neutrophil-mediated pulmonary vascular injury in endotoxemic pigs [65].

Other Models

Heparin-coated circuits were found to reduce complement activation and neutrophil and monocyte activation, e.g., cytokine and tissue factor release, and improve postoperative clinical performance after cardiac surgery involving cardiopulmonary bypass [66, 67]. Moreover, in experimental models of extracorporeal circulation, heparin coating inhibited the increase in leukocyte adhesion molecules, strongly correlated with inhibited complement activation and neutrophil degranulation [68, 69]. Finally, heparin pretreatment has been shown to prevent organ dysfunction and death in animals with I/R following hemorrhagic shock and resuscitation [70].

Fibrinolysis Activators

Recently, the effect of plasminogen activator on neutrophilic inflammation was also evaluated using the carrageenan-induced rat footpad inflammation model [71]. The administration of plasminogen activator inhibited, and streptokinase enhanced, inflammation. In some cases with fulminant meningococcemia, the administration of recombinant tissue plasminogen activator has resulted in improvement in organ perfusion and cardiac performance [72, 73].

Conclusion

Various data from experimental and clinical studies have accumulated showing a potential modulation by coagulation/fibrinolysis of the inflammatory response to sepsis and shock, so that anticoagulants may exert antiinflammatory effects independently of amelioration of the procoagulant/hypofibrinolytic state. These data may lead to a better understanding of the complex pathophysiological interaction between inflammation and coagulation and may also open new ways for the treatment of sepsis and shock. Future clinical trials to prove a beneficial effect of anticoagulants in these conditions might include assessment of antiinflammatory responses.

References

1. Groeneveld AB, Kindt I, Raijmakers PGHM, Hack CE, Thijs LG (1997) Systemic coagulation and fibrinolysis in patients with or at risk for the adult respiratory distress syndrome. Thromb Haemost 78:1444–1449
2. Vervloet MG, Thijs LG, Hack CE (1998) Derangements of coagulation and fibrinolysis in critically ill patients with sepsis and septic shock. Semin Thromb Hemost 24:33–44
3. Wu H-F, Lundblad RL, Church FC (1995) Neutralization of heparin activity by neutrophil lactoferrin. Blood 85:421–428

4. Sheu JR, Hung WC, Kan YC, Lee YM, Yen MH (1998) Mechanisms involved in the antiplatelet activity of Escherichia coli lipopolysaccharide in human platelets. Br J Haematol 103:29–38
5. Gerlach M, Keh D, Bezold G, Spielmann S, Kürer I, Peter RU, Falke KJ, Gerlach H (1998) Nitric oxide inhibits tissue factor synthesis, expression, and activity in human monocytes by prior formation of peroxynitrite. Intensive Care Med 24:1199–1208
6. Jourdain M, Tournoys A, Leroy X, Mangalaboyi J, Fourrier F, Goudemand J, Gosselin B, Vallet B, Chopin C (1997) Effects of N-$^{\Omega}$-nitro-L-arginine methyl ester on the endotoxin-induced disseminated intravascular coagulation in porcine septic shock. Crit Care Med 25:452–459
7. Ostrovsky L, Woodman RC, Payne D, Teoh D, Kubes P (1997) Antithrombin III prevents and rapidly reverses leukocyte recruitment in ischemia/reperfusion. Circulation 96: 2302–2310
8. Drake WT, Lopes NN, Fenton JW, Issekutz AC (1992) Thrombin enhancement of interleukin-1 and tumor necrosis factor-αinduced polymorphonuclear leukocyte migration. Lab Invest 67:617–627
9. Johnson L, Aarden L, Choi Y, De Groot E, Creasey A (1996) The proinflammatory cytokine response to coagulation and endotoxin in whole blood. Blood 87:5051–5060
10. Hébert CA, Luscinskas FW, Kiely J-M, Luis EA, Darbonne WC, Bennett GL, Liu CC, Obin MS, Gimbrone MA, Baker JB (1990) Endothelial and leukocyte forms of IL-8. Conversion by thrombin and interactions with neutrophils. J Immunol 145:3033–304
11. Mileno MD, Margolis NH, Clark BD, Dinarello CA, Burke JF, Gelfand JA (1995) Coagulation of whole blood stimulates interleukin-1 gene expression. J Infect Dis 172:308–311
12. Engstad CS, Guttebeberg TJ, Østerud B (1997) Modulation of blood cell activation by four commonly used anticoagulants. Thromb Haemost 77:690–696
13. Perez RL, Roman J (1995) Fibrin enhances the expression of IL-1β by human peripheral blood mononuclear cells. Implications in pulmonary inflammation. J Immunol 154: 1879–1887
14. Qi J, Kreutzer DL (1995) Fibrin activation of vascular endothelial cells. J Immunol 155: 867–876
15. Higazi AA, Barghouti II, Ayesh SK, Mayer M, Matzner Y (1994) Inhibition of neutrophil activation by fibrinogen. Inflammation 18:525–535
16. Robson SC, Shephard EG, Kirch RE (1994) Fibrin degradation product D-dimer induces the synthesis and release of biologically active IL-1β, IL-6 and plasminogen activator inhibitor from monocytes in vitro. Br J Haematol 86:322–326
17. Weyrich AS, Elstad MR, McEver RP, McIntyre TM, Moore KL, Morrissey JH, Prescott SM, Zimmerman GA (1996) Activated platelets signal chemokine synthesis by human monocytes. J Clin Invest 97:1525–1534
18. Gawaz M, Dickfeld T, Bogner C, Fateh-Maghadam S, Neumann FJ (1997). Platelet function in septic multiple organ dysfunction syndrome. Intensive Care Med 23:379–385
19. Heffner JE (1997) Platelet-neutrophil interactions in sepsis – platelet guilt by association? Intensive Care Med 23:366–368
20. Barry OP, Praticò D, Savani RC, FitzGerald GA (1998) Modulation of monocyte-endothelial interactions by platelet microparticles. J Clin Invest 102:136–144
21. Ruf A, Schlenk RF, Maras A, Morgenstern E, Patscheke H (1992) Contact-induced neutrophil activation by platelets in human cell suspensions and whole blood. Blood 80: 1–1246

22. Ruf A, Patscheke H (1995) Platelet-induced neutrophil activation: platelet-expressed fibrinogen induces the oxidative burst of neutrophils by an interaction with CD11 C/CD18 Br J Haematol 90:791–796
23. Hawrylowicz CM, Santoro SA, Platt FM, Unanue ER (1989) Activated platelets express IL-1 activity. J Immunol 143:4018
24. Kaplanski G, Porat R, Aiura K, Erban JK, Gelfand JA, Dinarello CA (1993) Activated platelets induce endothelial secretion of interleukin-8 in vitro via an interleukin-1-mediated event. Blood 81:2492–2495
25. Taylor FB, Chang ACK, Peer GT, Mather T, Blick K, Catlett R, Lockhart MS, Esmon CT (1991) DEGR-Factor Xa blocks disseminated intravascular coagulation by Escherichia coli without preventing shock or organ damage. Blood 78:364–368
26. Uchiba M, Okajima K, Murakami K, Nawa K, Okabe H, Takatsuki K (1995) Recombinant human soluble thrombomodulin reduces endotoxin-induced pulmonary vascular injury via protein C activation in rats. Thromb Haemost 74:1265–1270
27. Murakami K, Okajima K, Uchiba M, Johno M, Nakagaki T, Okabe H, Takatsuki K (1996) Activated protein C attenuates endotoxin-induced pulmonary vascular injury by inhibiting activated leukocytes in rats. Blood 87:642–647
28. Taylor FB, Chang A, Ruf W, Morrisey JH, Hinshaw L, Catlett R, Blick K, Edgington TS (1991) Lethal E. coli septic shock is prevented by blocking tissue factor with monoclonal antibody. Circ Shock 33:127–134
29. Dackiw APB, McGilvray ID, Woodside M, Nathens AB, Marshall JC, Rotstein OD (1996) Prevention of endotoxin-induced mortality by antitissue factor immunization. Arch Surg 131:1273–1279
30. Levi M, Ten Cate H, Bauer KA, Van der Poll T, Edgington TS, Büller HR, Van Deventer SJH, Hack CE, Tan Cate JW, Rosenberg RD (1994) Inhibition of endotoxin-induced activation of coagulation and fibrinolysis by pentoxifylline or by a monoclonal anti-tissue factor antibody in chimpanzees. J Clin Invest 93:114–120
31. Creasey AA, Chang ACK, Feigen L, Wün T-C, Taylor FB, Hinshaw LB (1993) Tissue factor pathway inhibitor reduces mortality from Escherichia coli septic shock. J Clin Invest 91:2850–2860
32. Carr C, Bild GS, Chang ACK, Peer GT, Palmier MO, Frazxier RB, Gustafson ME, Wun T-C, Creasey AA, Hinshaw LB, Taylor FB, Gallupi GR (1995) Recombinant E. coli-derived tissue factor pathway inhibitor reduces coagulopathic and lethal effects in the baboon gram-negative model of septic shock. Circ Shock 44:126–137
33. Park CT, Creasey AA, Wright SD (1997) Tissue factor pathway inhibitor blocks cellular effects of endotoxin by binding endotoxin and interfering with transfer to CD14. Blood 89:4268–4274
34. Taylor FB, Chang A, Esmon CT, D'Angelo A, Vigano-D'Angelo S, Blick KE. (1987) Protein C prevents the coagulopathic and lethal effects of Escherichia coli infusion in the baboon. J Clin Invest 79:918–925
35. Takahashi Y, Hosaka Y, Imada K, Adachi T, Niina H, Watanabe M, Mochizuki H (1997) Human urinary soluble thrombomodulin (MR-33) improves disseminated intravascular coagulation without affecting bleeding time in rats: comparison with low-molecular-weight heparin. Thromb Haemost 77:789–795
36. Grey ST, Hannock WW (1996) A physiologic anti-inflammatory pathway based on thrombomodulin expression and generation of activated protein C by human mononuclear phagocytes. J Immunol 156:2256–2263

37. Grey ST, Tsuchida A, Hau H, Orthner CL, Salem HH, Hancock WW (1994) Selective inhibitory effects of the anticoagulant activated protein C on the responses of human mononuclear phagocytes to LPS, IFN-gamma, or phorbol ester. J Immunol 153: 3664–3672
38. Fourrier F, Jourdain M, Tournoys A, Gosset P, Mangalaboyi J, Chopin C (1998) Effects of a combined antithrombin III and protein C supplementation in porcine acute endotoxic shock. Shock 10:364–370
39. Gerson WT, Dickerman JD, Bovill EG, Golden E (1993) Severe acquired protein C deficiency in purpura fulminans associated with disseminated intravascular coagulation: treatment with protein C concentrate. Pediatrics 91:418–422
40. Rivard G, Dvid M, Farrelll C, Schwarz HP (1995) Treatment of purpura fulminans in meningococcemia with protein C concentrate. J Pediatr 126:646–652
41. Triantahyllopoulos DC (1984) Effects of human antithrombin III on mortality and blood coagulation induced in rabbits by endotoxin. Thromb Haemost 51:232–235
42. Taylor FB, Emerson TE, Jordan R, Chang AK, Blick KE (1988) Antithrombin III prevents the lethal effects of Escherichia coli infusion in baboons. Circ Shock 26:227–235
43. Kessler CM, Tang ZC, Jacobs HM, Szymanski KM (1997) The suprapharmacologic dosing of antithrombin concentrate for Staphylococcus aureus-induced disseminated intravascular coagulation in guinea pigs: substantial reduction in mortality and morbidity. Blood 89:4393–4401
44. Yamanuchi T, Umeda F, Inoguchi T, Nawata H (1989) Antithrombin III stimulates prostacyclin production by cultured aortic endothelial cells. Biochem Biophys Res Commun 163:1404–1411
45. Uchiba M, Okajima K, Murakami K, Okade H, Takatsuki K (1995) Effect of antithrombin III (ATIII) and TRP49-modified AT III on plasma levels of 6-keto-$PGF_{1\alpha}$ in rats. Thromb Res 80:201–208
46. Uchiba M, Okajima K, Murakami K, Okade H, Takatsuki K (1996) Attenuation of endotoxin induced pulmonary vascular injury by antithrombin III. Am J Physiol 270:L921–L930
47. Uchiba M, Okajima K, Murakami K (1998) Effects of various doses of antithrombin III on endotoxin-induced endothelial cell injury and coagulation abnormalities in rats. Thromb Res 89:233–241
48. Emerson TE (1994) Antithrombin III replacement in animal models of acquired antithrombin III deficiency Blood Coag Fibrinolysis 5:S37-S45
49. Jochum M (1995) Influence of high dose antithrombin concentrate therapy on the release of cellular proteinases, cytokines and soluble adhesion molecules in acute inflammation. Semin Hematol 32 [Suppl 2]:19–32
50. Inthorn D, Hoffmann JN, Hartl WH, Mühlbayer D, Jochum M (1998) Effect of antithrombin III supplementation on inflammatory response in patients with severe sepsis. Shock 10:90–96
51. Eisele B, Lamy M, Thijs LG, Keinecke H-O, Schuster H-P, Matthias FR, Fourrier F, Heinrichs H, Delvos U (1998) Antithrombin III in patients with severe sepsis. A randomized, placebo-controlled, double-blind multicenter trial plus a metanalysis on all randomized, placebo-controlled, doubleblind trials with AIII in severe sepsis. Intens Care Med 24:663–672
52. Baudo F, Caimi TM, deCataldo F, Ravizza A, Arlati S, Casella G, Carugo D, Palareti G, Legnani C, Ridolfi L, Rossi R, D'Angelo A, Crippa L, Giudici D, Gallioli G, Wolfler A, Calori G (1998) Antithrombin III (ATIII) replacement therapy in patients with sepsis

and/or postsurgical complications: a controlled double-blind, randomized, multicenter study. Intens Care Med 24:336–342
53. Harada N, Okajima K, Kushomoto S, Isobe H, Tanaka K (1999) Antithrombin reduces ischemia/reperfusion injury of rat liver by increasing the hepatic level of prostacyclin. Blood 93:157–164
54. Bleeker WK, Agterberg J, Rigter G, Hack CE, Gool JV (1992) Protective effect of antithrombin III in acute experimental pancreatitis in rats. Dig Dis Sci 37:280–285
55. Yamaguchi H, Weindebach H, Luchrs H, Lerch MM, Dickneite G, Adler G (1997) Combined treatment with C1 esterase inhibitor and antithrombin III improves survival in severe acute experimental pancreatitis. Gut 40:531–535
56. Høgasen AKM, Abrahamsen TG (1995) Heparin increases lipopolysaccharide-induced monocyte production of several cytokines, but simultanesouly stimulates C3 production. Thromb Res 80:179–184
57. Attanasio M, Gori AM, Giusti B, Pepe G, Comeglio P, Brunelli T, Prisco D, Abbate R, Gensini GF, Neri Serneri GG (1998) Cytokine gene expression in human LPS- and INF-gamma-stimulated mononuclear cells is inhibited by heparin. Thromb Haemost 79: 959–962
58. Call DR, Remick DG (1998) Low-molecular-weight heparin is associated with greater cytokine production in a stimulated whole blood model. Shock 10:192–197
59. El Habbal MH, Smith L, Elliott MJ, Strobel S (1995) Effect of heparin anticoagulation on neutrophil adhesion molecules and release of IL-8: C3 is not essential. Cardiovasc Res 30:676–681
60. Miller SJ, Hoggat AM, Faulk WP (1998) Heparin regulates ICAM-1 expression in human endothelial cells: an example of non cytokine-mediated endothelial activation. Thromb Haemost 80:481–487
61. Webb LMC, Ehrengruber MU, Clark-Lewis I, Baggioni M, Rot A (1993) Binding to heparan sulfate or heparin enhances neutrophil responses to interleukin 8. Proc Natl Acad Sci USA 90:7158–7162
62. Lantz M, Thysell H, Nilsson E, Olsson I (1991) On the binding of tumor necrosis factor (TNF) to heparin and the release in vivo of the TNF-binding protein I by heparin. J Clin Invest 88:2026–2031
63. Moulin F, Pearson JM, Schultze AE, Scott MA, Schwartz KA, Davis JM, Gancey PE, Roth RA (1996) Thrombin is a distal mediator of lipopolysacchardie-induced liver injury in the rat. J Surg Res 65:149–158
64. Morrison AM, Wang P, Chaudry IH (1996) A novel nonanticoagulant heparin prevents vascular endothelial dysfunction during hyperdynamic sepsis. Shock 6:46–51
65. Darien BJ, Fareed J, Centgraf KS, Hart AP, MacWIlliams PS, Clayton MK, Wolf H, Kruse-Elliott KT (1998) Low molecular weight heparin prevents the pulmonary hemodynamic and pathomorphologic effects of endotoxin in a porcine acute lung injury model. Shock 9:274–281
66. Jansen PGM, Te Velthuis H, Huibregts RAJM, Paulus R, Bulder ER, Van der Spoel HI, Bezemer PD, Slaats EH, Eijsman L, Wildevuur CRH (1995) Reduced complement activation and improved postoperative performance after cardiopulmonary bypass with heparin-coated circuits. J Thorac Cardiovasc Surg 110:829–843
67. Baufreton C, Moczar M, Intrator L, Jansen PG, te Velthuis H, Besnerais PL, Farcet JP, Wildevuur CR, Loisance DY (1998) Inflammatory response to cardiopulmonary bypass using two different types of heparin-coated extracorporeal circuits. Perfusion 13:419–427

68. Garred P, Molness TE (1997) Immobilized heparin inhibits the increase in leukocyte surface expression of adhesion molecules. Artif Organs 21:293–239
69. Hogevold HE, Moen O, Fosse E, Venge P, Braten J, Andersson C, Lyberg T (1997) Effects of heparin coating on the expression of CD11b, CD11 C and CD62L by leukocytes in extracorpopreal circulation in vitro. Perfusion 12:9–20
70. Wang P, Singh G, Rana MW, Ba ZF, Chaudry IH (1990) Preheparinizaton improves organ function after hemorrhage and resuscitation. Am J Physiol 259:R645-R650
71. Stringer KA, Bose SK, McCord JM (1997) Antiinflammatory activity of tissue plasminogen activator in the carrageenan rat footpad model. Free Radic Biol Med 22(6):985–988
72. Zenz W, Muntean W, Gallistl S, Zobel G, Grubbauer HM (1995) Recombinant tissue plasminogen activator treatment in two infants with fulminant meningococcemia. Pediatrics 96:144–148
73. Aiuto LT, Barone SR, Cohen PS, Boxer RA (1997) Recombinant tissue plasminogen activator restores perfusion in meningococcal purpura fulminans. Crit Care Med 25: 1079–1082

Normalization of Plasma Antithrombin Activity in Patients Requiring Hemodynamic and/or Respiratory Support has Anti-inflammatory Properties Related to Survival

A. D'Angelo, P. Della Valle, C. Legnani , G. Palareti, A. Ravizza, L. Ridolfi, D. Giudici, F. Baudo, and S. Kurosawa

The Italian Antithrombin Sepsis Study has shown that maintenance of antithrombin (AT) levels around 100% results in a 53% reduction in the 30-day mortality risk of intensive care unit patients with sepsis and/or post-surgical complications requiring hemodynamic and/or respiratory support [1, 2]. The changes in a series of coagulation and fibrinolysis parameters were evaluated with the aim of correlating such changes with the potential effect of AT treatment on survival and exploring the predictive value of laboratory tests on 30-day mortality [3]. Blood samples from 119 patients were taken at baseline and then daily until day 7 from the beginning of AT or placebo infusion. The parameters evaluated were: AT activity, protein C (PC) and S activity and antigen levels, α_2-antiplasmin and plasminogen activity, fibrin and fibrinogen degradation products, plasmin–antiplasmin complex, prothrombin fragment 1.2, and thrombin–antithrombin (TAT) complex. Prealbumin was also measured to correct for impaired liver synthesis of coagulation and fibrinolysis factors and inhibitors. Improvement – but never normalization – in most of the laboratory parameters was observed over time. In addition to AT, treatment only affected TAT levels ($p=0.05$). In a Cox survival regression model, including the presence of septic shock, the multiorgan failure (MOF) score and the type of treatment as covariates, baseline AT levels were an independent predictor of mortality in the entire series of patients ($p=0.003$). After 24 h of treatment, TAT levels were negatively associated with survival ($p=0.05$). On the last day of treatment, the levels of PC ($p=0.006$) and of fibrinogen-degradation products ($p=0.005$) were negatively and positively associated with mortality in the 91 survivors [3].

Antithrombin inhibits coagulation factors generated in the coagulation cascade. The inhibition of proteases by AT is markedly accelerated by its interaction with glycosaminoglycans on the endothelial cell surface [4]. Prostacyclin is a well-known cytoprotective agent that is synthesized in endothelial cells [5]. AT promotes the endothelial release of prostacyclin in vitro and in vivo by interacting with cell surface glycosaminoglycans [6, 7]. In addition to vasodilatation,

PGI_2 inhibits leukocyte activation by inhibiting tumor necrosis factor α production by monocytes [8], neutrophil activation [9], and neutrophil adhesion to endothelial cells [10]. Because activated leukocytes release a variety of inflammatory mediators, including cytokines, neutrophil proteases, and reactive oxygen species, all of which can damage adjacent endothelial cells, they have been thought to play a pivotal role in tissue injury [11–17]. AT supplementation was shown to reduce mortality in animals challenged with lipopolysaccharide or *Escherichia coli* [18], and to increase the survival rate of rabbits exposed to LPS without improving coagulopathy [19]. These observations suggest that the beneficial effects of AT in sepsis may be due to both its anticoagulant activity and another unknown action. AT prevents endotoxin-induced pulmonary vascular injury by promoting PGI2 release from endothelial cells, independent of its anticoagulant activity [20]. Similar results were obtained in a rat model of liver ischemia–reperfusion injury, still pointing to an effect mediated by the endogenous release of prostacyclin [21]. Because PGI2 inhibits the production of TNF, which enhances the production of IL-8, a potent activator of neutrophils [22, 23], it is possible that AT may also prevent ischemia–reperfusion injury in rats by inhibiting leukocyte activation through the promotion of PGI2 production. However, in hepatic injury induced by ischemia–reperfusion of whole liver rats, AT has been shown to prevent hepatic injury by inhibiting coagulation abnormalities [24]. Thus, it is possible that AT can prevent ischemia–reperfusion-induced hepatic injury by inhibiting thrombin activity as well as by inhibiting leukocyte activation through the induction of PGI2 release. Jochum has demonstrated that infusion of AT concentrate significantly inhibits hepatic dysfunction in patients with multiple traumas by inhibiting leukocyte activation [25]. This author infused high-dose antithrombin concentrate, aiming at plasma levels similar to those attained by Fourrier et al. in their study of septic shock patients [26].

An ancillary study evaluated in a subgroup of 24 patients enrolled in the Italian Antithrombin Sepsis Study the potential effect of AT supplementation on mediators of the inflammatory response, on soluble adhesion molecules, and on soluble markers of endothelial cell activation/damage.

Materials and Methods

The design, inclusion and exclusion criteria, and treatment schedules of the Italian AT sepsis study have been previously reported. Patients enrolled were sampled on each day for 7 days. Venous blood was drawn before administration of the bolus dose of AT or placebo, 30 min after the bolus dose, and then daily for 2 additional days after interruption of treatment. All samples were collected between 8:00 and 10:30 A.M. in silicone pirogen-free vacutainer tubes containing 0.129 mol/l sodium citrate (Becton Dickinson, 1/10 blood volume) or in Bauer's anticoagulant. Platelet poor plasma was obtained by centrifugation at room temperature at 3000 *g* for 15 min within 45 min from blood drawing. Plasma aliquots were snap-frozen in methanol and dry ice and stored at –70 °C until assay. The investigation reported in this paper involved 24 patients (18 men and five women, mean age 62.6±11.8 years), all recruited in one center (H S. Raffaele, Milano), who had survived the first week of observation. Nine patients required hemodynamic and/or respiratory support because of post-surgical complications; five patients had sepsis and ten had septic shock, as defined in accordance with the guidelines of the American College of Chest Physicians/Society of Critical Care Medicine consensus conference [27]. Fourteen patients received treatment with AT and ten with placebo. Thirty-day mortality was 67% (6/9) in sepsis-free patients, 60% (3/5) in patients with sepsis, and 70% (7/10) in patients with septic shock. In this subgroup of patients, 30-day mortality was not significantly different in patients receiving AT (78%, 11/14) or placebo (50%, 5/10, Fisher's exact test, $p=0.15$).

Laboratory Methods

Human tumor necrosis factor α (TNF-α), interleukin-1β (IL-1β), IL-4, IL-6, IL-8 and IL-10 were measured by ELISA (EASIA-kit) with kits purchased from Medgenix Diagnostics (Fleurus, Belgium). Human soluble E-selectin (sCD62E) and vascular cell adhesion molecule-1 (sVCAM-1) were measured by ELISA kits purchased from Endogen (Woburn, MA, USA) and Biosource International (Camarillo, CA, USA). Polymorphonuclear elastase (PMN elastase) was measured by tubidimetry with the Hitachi 717 analyzer (Boehringer Mannheim, Germany) according to the instructions provided by the manufacturer (Ecoline PMN Elastase, Merck KgaA, Darmstadt, Germany). The soluble endothelial protein C receptor (sEPCR) was measured as previously described [28]. But for sEPCR, all measurements were performed in duplicate in a single laboratory (H S. Raffaele). For each patient, samples drawn at baseline, on day 2 of treatment and on day 6 (one day after the end of treatment) were analyzed for all of the above parameters.

Statistical Analysis

For descriptive purposes, results are expressed as mean value ± standard deviation (SD). Because normal distributions were not obtained by log-transformation of data, rank-transformation of data was adopted. One-way analysis of variance (ANOVA) and ANOVA for repeated measures were used to compare continuous variables among the groups of patients. The Spearman test was used to correlate the parameters evaluated. For multiple comparisons, p values were corrected according to Bonferroni's procedure. Proportions were analyzed by the χ^2 test or the Fisher's exact test. The Systat® statistical software program was used for all calculations.

Results

Table 1 reports the plasma levels at baseline of the cytokines, of PMN elastase, of the soluble adhesion molecules and of soluble EPCR according to the presence of sepsis and/or septic shock. The percentage of patients with levels higher than the upper limit of the normal range (as reported by the manufacturers) is also shown. With the exception of IL-10 and sCD62E, marked elevations in the parameters evaluated were observed in all patients irrespective of the presence of sepsis and/or septic shock. TNF-α levels were higher in patients with septic shock than in patients with sepsis ($p=0.05$). A trend was observed for IL-10 levels to be higher in patients with sepsis and/or septic shock than in the remaining patients ($p=0.059$), and the proportion of patients with sepsis and/or septic shock with abnormally elevated levels (53%) was greater than that of patients without sepsis (11%, $p=0.039$). IL-6, sCD62E and PMN elastase levels differed in the three groups of patients, with the higher levels detected in patients with septic shock. IL-8 levels were higher in patients with septic shock ($p=0.043$). sCD62E levels were higher in patients with sepsis and/or septic shock ($p=0.037$), but abnormal sCD62E elevations were only observed in sepsis complicated by shock ($p=0.01$).

When related to 30-day mortality, no variable at baseline distinguished eventually deceased patients from survivors. However, sCD62E baseline levels were higher in patients treated with AT than with placebo (20.2 ± 10.4 vs. 11.4 ± 4.5 ng/ml, $p=0.008$).

Changes in the parameters with time were analyzed by univariate and multivariate repeated measures analysis, as a function of the presence of sepsis

Table 1. Baseline levels of cytokines, PMN elastase, soluble adhesion molecules and endothelial protein C receptor (mean ± SD) and percentage of patients with values higher than the upper limit of the normal range according to the presence of sepsis and/or septic shock

	Normal values[a]	No sepsis ($n=9$)		Sepsis ($n=5$)		Septic shock $n=10$)		p-Value	
	Mean ± SD	Mean ± SD	Percentage	Mean ± SD	Percentage	Mean ± SD	Percentage	ANOVA on ranked data	χ^2 for proportions
TNF-α (pg/ml)	6.0 ± 4.0	63.9 ± 36.0	89	53.8 ± 17.8	100	85.4 ± 38.7	100	ns	ns
IL-1β (pg/ml)	5.0 ± 8.0	16.4 ± 5.3	56	10.3 ± 7.2	40	15.3 ± 7.2	70	ns	ns
IL-4 (pg/ml)	1.6 ± 2.1	10.5 ± 1.2	100	9.7 ± 0.3	100	10.3 ± 0.8	100	ns	ns
IL-6 (pg/ml)	<3.0	205.4 ± 80.1	100	771.1 ± 662.8	100	2056.7 ± 2609.0	100	0.002	ns
IL-8 (pg/ml)	8.0 ± 10.0	60.3 ± 33.6	78	98.8 ± 88.7	100	174.0 ± 217.6	100	ns	ns
IL-10 (pg/ml)	2.5 ± 3.2	4.3 ± 5.1	11	11.2 ± 7.3	60	20.1 ± 24.4	50	ns	ns
PMN elastase (ng/ml)	22 ± 20	149.6 ± 46.5	78	166.6 ± 38.3	100	263.0 ± 53.6	100	0.001	ns
sCD62E (ng/ml)	16.9 ± 5.4	11.9 ± 5.8	0	14.1 ± 2.6	0	21.9 ± 11.7	50	0.047	0.012
sVCAM-1 (ng/ml)	550 ± 105	2441 ± 1103	89	3683 ± 2399	60	2000 ± 1130	90	ns	ns
sEPCR (ng/ml)	133.4 ± 53.4	187.8 ± 66.6	22	254.7 ± 83.8	60	224.0 ± 70.2	20	ns	ns

[a] As reported by the manufacturers or as established in 18 normal volunteers for sEPCR

and/or septic shock, outcome at 30 days, and treatment. Changes in TNF-α, IL-6, IL-10 and PMN elastase plasma levels are reported in Fig. 1. Significant changes in TNF-α levels were observed over time ($p=0.025$), with changes differing significantly according to the presence of septic shock ($p=0.0001$) and outcome ($p=0.02$). In patients with septic shock and unfavorable outcome there was no change in TNF-α levels with time, whereas TNF-α levels decreased to about 50% of baseline levels by day 6 in survivors with septic shock. IL-6 levels decreased with time in patients with septic shock, but the rate of decrease was faster in survivors than in non-survivors ($p=0.08$). IL-10 levels decreased with time to a significantly greater extent in survivors than in non-survivors ($p=0.014$), and especially so in patients with septic shock ($p=0.08$). The presence of septic shock was consistently associated with higher circulating levels of PMN elastase ($p=$

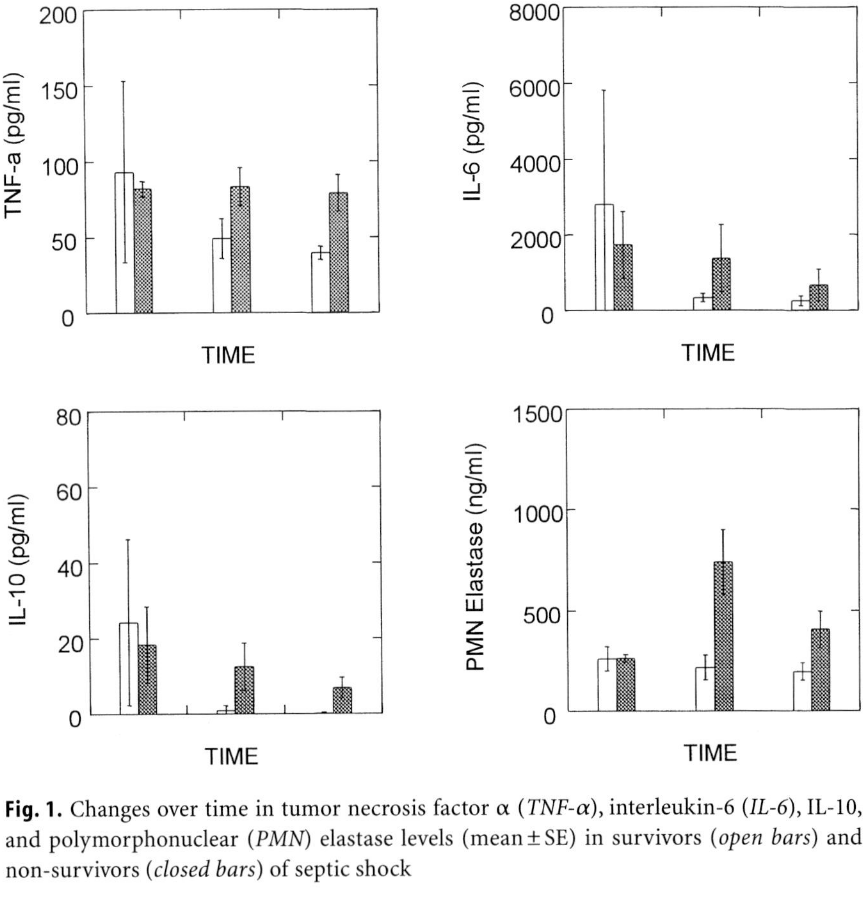

Fig. 1. Changes over time in tumor necrosis factor α (*TNF-α*), interleukin-6 (*IL-6*), IL-10, and polymorphonuclear (*PMN*) elastase levels (mean ± SE) in survivors (*open bars*) and non-survivors (*closed bars*) of septic shock

0.020). PMN elastase levels were unchanged in survivors with septic shock, but they increased significantly in non-survivors with septic shock ($p = 0.040$).

IL-8 levels decreased with time in all patients, but the decrease was greater in survivors than in non-survivors ($p = 0.021$), irrespective of the presence of septic shock (Fig. 2). IL-8 levels were lower in patients receiving AT than in those receiving placebo ($p = 0.047$). sCD62E levels changed with time as a function of outcome and treatment ($p = 0.027$). AT supplementation led to a decrease in sCD62E levels in both survivors and non-survivors. In contrast, non-survivors receiving placebo showed an increase in sCD62E levels (Fig. 2).

IL-1β, IL-4, VCAM-1 and sEPCR levels did not show significant changes.

Statistically significant, positive correlations were observed at baseline between TNF-α and IL-10 levels ($\varrho = 0.635, p = 0.045$), IL-10 and IL-6 levels ($\varrho = 0.650, p = 0.032$). On day 2 of treatment TNF-α levels were strongly correlated to

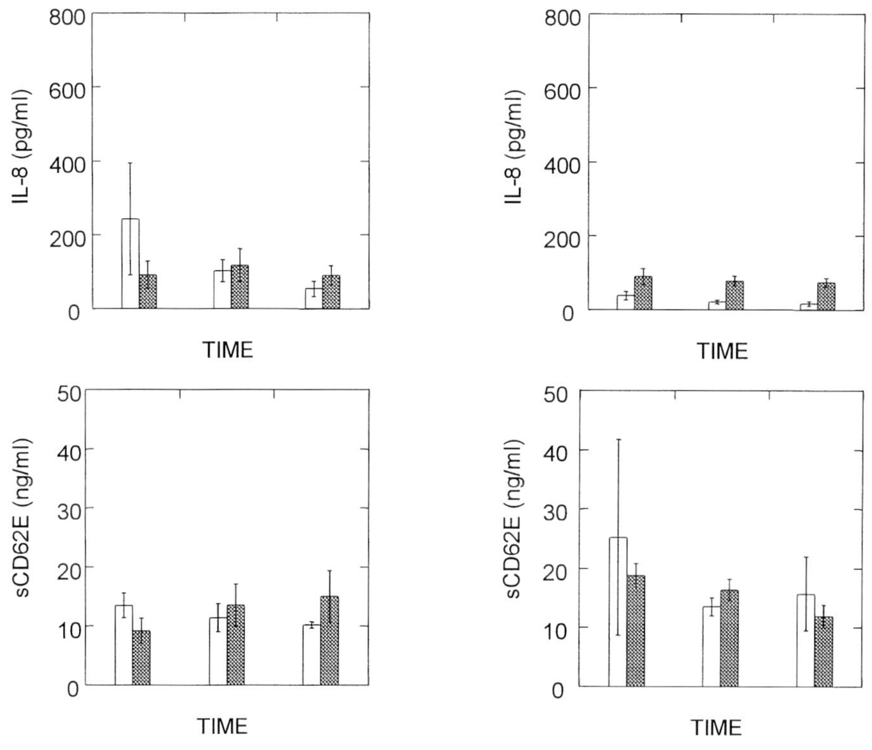

Fig. 2. Changes over time in interleukin-8 (IL-8) and sCD62E plasma levels (mean ± SE) according to outcome (survivors, *open bars*; non-survivors, *closed bars*) in patients receiving placebo (left panels) or antithrombin (right panels)

IL-10 levels ($\varrho = 0.730$, $p = 0.003$). On day 6 there was no significant correlation among the parameters evaluated.

On day 6, higher levels of TNF-α ($p = 0.046$), IL-8 ($p = 0.003$) and IL-10 ($p = 0.031$) were associated with unfavorable patients' outcome irrespective of the presence of septic shock at baseline. Higher PMN elastase levels were associated with unfavorable outcome only in patients with septic shock ($p = 0.029$). IL-8 levels were lower in patients who had received AT than in those who had been infused with placebo ($p = 0.029$).

Discussion

TNF-α is mainly produced by activated monocytes and is an important mediator of the inflammatory response. In addition to antitumoral and growth regulatory activity, it activates macrophages, neutrophils and eosinophils, as well as endothelial cells, which display procoagulant activity. Besides the involvement in the humoral and cellular immune response, TNF-α induces the production of additional mediators of inflammation, such as IL-1, IL-6, prostaglandins, platelet activating factor etc. [29]. In septic shock, neutralization of TNF-α protects against the associated acute lethality [30], and TNF-α levels may have prognostic significance [31]. IL-1 is a key mediator of the host response to various infections, and to inflammatory and immunological challenges [32]. Levels of IL-1 plasma are mainly regulated by its production by blood monocytes and tissue macrophages, but other cell types (for instance endothelial cells) may also produce IL-1. IL-1β is the major IL-1 form in circulating plasma [33]. IL-1 affects several unrelated tissues and has en essential role in T-cell activation [34]. It is the main mediator of inflammatory processes due to its action on the nervous system, on bone marrow-derived cells, and on various tissues (stimulation of endothelial cell procoagulant activity). Most of these activities are directly attributable to IL-1β, but others are mediated in collaboration with other cytokines such as IL-6, interferons, and TNF. IL-1 stimulates the production of or acts sinergistically with these cytokines, and the final biological activity is the result of a network of interactions between these various mediators [35]. Although little or no IL-1β is normally detected in human plasma from healthy, rested subjects, elevated levels have been reported in the circulation of septic patient [36]. IL-6 is produced by various cells, including lymphocytes, monocytes and endothelial cells, and regulates the growth and differentiation of various cell types with major activities on the immune system, hematopoiesis and inflammation. It promotes megakaryocyte development and is a major inducer of the acute phase reactions in response to inflammation or tissue injury. Along with IL-1 and TNF, it induces the synthesis of acute phase proteins by hepatocytes, each cytokine or combination of cytokines showing a preferential pattern of acute phase protein production. Although most normal controls have undetectable levels of IL-6 in their plasma, huge quantities of IL-6 are detected in severe inflammatory situations such as septicemia [37]. IL-8 is a chemoattractant protein for neutrophils. Different cells such as monocytes, neutrophils, and endothelial cells etc. [38] secrete this pro-inflammatory mediator. The IL-8 level in septic shock patients was found to correlate with mortality [39]. In contrast to the above cytokines, IL-4 and IL-10 have anti-inflammatory properties. IL-4 is produced by the TH2 subtype of CD4+ T-lymphocytes and by mast cell precursors. IL-4 blocks the production of IL-1, IL-6 TNF-α, PGE2, G-CSF and stimulates the production of M-CSF and G-CSF by the monocytes [40]. IL-4 can augment the capacity of TNF-α to selectively promote VCAM-1 expression [41]. T-helper lymphocytes, monocytes, macrophages and B-lymphocytes produce IL-10. IL-10 specifically inhibits IL-2 production by responding T-cells. In vitro, IL-10 is a very powerful inhibitor of TNF-α, IL-1, IL-6 and IL-8 produced by LPS-activated monocytes and macrophages [42]. Natural killer cells are presumably another target for the anti-inflammatory properties of IL-10. Circulating levels of IL-10 have been found in patients suffering septic shock [43].

IL-1β and TNF-α induce new endothelial cell surface molecules during the initial phase of an inflammatory response. E-selectin (CD62E, ELAM-1) is a member of the family of structurally related molecules (selectins) that participate in endothelial–leukocyte adhesion [44]. E-selectin mediates the adhesion of polymorphonuclear cells, monocytes, and some memory T-cells to cytokine-activated endothelial cells. Venular and capillary endothelial cells at sites of active inflammation [45] express it. VCAM-1, a member of the immunoglobulin gene superfamily, is a cell surface adhesion molecule that mediates the adhesion of monocytes, lymphocytes, basophils and eosinophils (but not neutrophils) to human umbilical vein endothelial cells [46]. These two inducible endothelial adhesion molecules have distinct time courses of cytokine induction. In cultured human endothelial cells, CD62E first appears on the cell surface within 1–2 h of cytokine treatment [47]. Maximal expression occurs at 4–6 h and then rapidly declines in the continued presence of cytokine, reaching basal levels by 24 h. VCAM-1 first appears at 4–6 hours, reaches maximal levels at 12–18 h, and then gradually declines over several days [48]. In vivo studies have, however, shown a similar, more sustained expression of both adhesion molecules [49].

The endothelial protein C receptor (EPCR) is a recently described member of the protein C anticoagulant pathway [50, 51]. The membrane form of EPCR – expressed almost exclusively on the large vessels, but not in the microcirculation where thrombomodulin is abundant [52] – works in concert with thrombomodulin to augment protein C activation on endothelial cells [53], whereas a soluble form of EPCR from normal human plasma inhibits the generation and function of activated protein C [54].

In this study we investigated the relationship of changes in cytokines and soluble adhesion molecules with the presence of sepsis/and or septic shock, 30-day mortality and AT treatment in a subgroup of 24 patients enrolled in the Italian Antithrombin Sepsis Study. Although the evaluation included a relatively small number of patients, there was a clear association of baseline elevations in some of the parameters (TNF-α, IL-6, IL-8, IL-10, sCD62E, and PMN elastase) with septic shock. No parameter predicted 30-day mortality at baseline. However, changes in the levels of some of the parameters were associated with the patients' outcome when measured on days 2 and 6 after enrollment in the study. Thus, in patients with septic shock, TNF-α levels decreased in 30-day survivors, but they were unchanged in non-survivors, and the rate of decrease in IL-6 and IL-10 levels was faster in survivors than in nonsurvivors. Conversely, PMN elastase levels were unchanged in survivors with septic shock, but they showed a substantial increase in non-survivors with septic shock. The changes in IL-8 and sCD62E levels with time were not related to the presence of septic shock, but were associated with the patients' outcome, with non-survivors showing a lesser decrease (IL-8) or an increase in the circulating levels (sCD62E). The significance of these modifications was confirmed by the predictive value for unfavorable outcome associated with high levels of TNF-α, IL-8, IL-10 and PMN elastase measured on day 6.

Taken together, these data confirm the pathogenic role of pro-inflammatory cytokines in patients with sepsis. In addition, they strongly suggest that IL-8 and sCD62E levels may be useful for monitoring the severity of disease in sepsis-free patients admitted to the intensive care unit because of the need for hemodynamic and/or respiratory support.

The plasma levels of IL-8 and sCD62E were also influenced by antithrombin supplementation in patients. We show for the first time that a 5-day course of AT infusion aimed at maintaining plasma antithrombin activity at about 100% is effective in reducing IL-8 and sCD62E levels irrespective of the patients' outcome and of the presence of septic shock. Previous data had shown that AT has an effect on pro-inflammatory molecules only when it is administered at high dosages aimed at maintaining supernormal plasma antithrombin activity [25]. Taken together with the laboratory results previously reported from the Italian Antithrombin Sepsis Study, AT supplementation aimed at the normalization of plasma antithrombin activity modulates hypercoagulability/hyperfibrinolysis and displays anti-inflammatory properties, both participating in the beneficial effects on 30-day mortality of severely ill patients.

References

1. Baudo F, Caimi T, deCataldo F, Ravizza A, Arlati S, Casella G, Carugo D, Palareti G, Legnani C, Ridolfi L, Rossi R, D'Angelo A, Crippa L, Giudici D, Gallioli G, Wolfler A, Calori G (1998) Antithrombin III (AT III) replacement therapy in patients with sepsis and/or postsurgical complications: a controlled double blind, randomized multicenter study. Intensive Care Med 24:336
2. Giudici D, Ravizza A, Ridolfi L, Baudo F, Palareti G, D'Angelo A (1999) Antithrombin replacement in patients with sepsis and septic shock. Haematologica 84:452
3. D'Angelo A, Palareti G (1996) The italian antithrombin III sepsis study: laboratory aspects. Second International Winter Meeting on Coagulation: Basic, Laboratory and Clinical Aspects of Thromboembolic Diseases. La Thuile, Italy. (Abstract 25)
4. Rosenberg RD (1989) Biochemistry of heparin antithrombin interactions, and the physiological role of this natural anticoagulant mechanisms. Am J Med 87:2 S [Suppl 3b]
5. Granger DN, Kubes P (1994) The microcirculation and inflammation: modulation of leukocyte-endothelial cell adhesion. J Leukoc Biol 55:662
6. Horie S, Ishii H, Kazama M (1990) Heparin-like glycosaminoglycan is a receptor for antithrombin III-dependent but not for thrombin-dependent prostacyclin production in human endothelial cells. Thromb Res 59:895
7. Yamauchi T, Umeda F, Inoguchi T, Nawata H (1989) Antithrombin III stimulates prostacyclin production by cultured aortic endothelial cells. Biochem Biophys Res Commun 163:1404
8. Eisenhut T, Shina B, Grottrup-Wolfers E, Semmler J, Siess W, Endres S (1993) Prostacyclin analogs suppress the synthesis of tumor necrosis factor-αa in LPS-stimulated human peripheral blood mononuclear cells. Immunopharmacology 26:259
9. Kainoh M, Imai R, Umetsu T, Hattori M, Nishio S (1990) Prostacyclin and beraprost sodium as suppressors of activated rat polymorphonuclear leukocytes. Biochem Pharmacol 39:477
10. Boxer LA, Allen JM, Schmidt M, Yoder M, Baehner RL (1990) Inhibition of polymorphonuclear leukocyte adherence by prostacyclin. J Lab Clin Med 95:672
11. Starkey PM (1977) Elastase and cathepsin G: the serine proteases of human neutrophil leukocytes and spleen. In: Barret AJ (ed) Proteinases in mammalian cells and tissues. Elsevier/North Holland, Amsterdam, p 57
12. Weiss SJ, LoBuglio AF (1980) An oxygen-dependent mechanism of neutrophil-mediated cytotoxicity. Blood 55:1020
13. Weiss SJ, Young J, LoBuglio AF, Slivka A, Nimeh NF (1981) Role of hydrogen peroxide in neutrophil-mediated destruction of cultured endothelial cells. J Clin Invest 68:714

14. Komatsu H, Koo A, Ghadishah E, Zeng H, Kuhlenkamp JF, Inoue M, Guth PH, Kaplowitz N (1992) Neutrophil accumulation in ischemic reperfused rat liver: evidence for a role for superoxide free radicals. Am J Physiol 262:G699
15. Jaeschke H, Bautista AP, Spolarics Z, Spitzer JJ (1992) Superoxide generation by neutrophils and kuppfer cells during in vivo reperfusion after hepatic ischemia in rats. J Leukoc Biol 52:377
16. Colleti LM, Burtch GD, Remick DG, Strieter RM, Guice KS, Oldham KT, Campbell DA Jr (1990) The production of tumor necrosis factor αa and the development of a pulmonary capillary injury following heaptic ischemia/reperfusion. Transplantation 49: 268
17. Shito M, Wakabayashi G, Ueda M, Shimazu M, Shirasugi N, Endo M, Mukai M, Kitajima M (1997) Interleukin 1 receptor blockade reduces tumor necrosis factor production, tissue injury, and mortality after hepatic iscehmia-reperfusion in the rat. Transplantation 63:143
18. Emerson TE, Fournel MA, Redens TB, Taylor FB (1989) Efficacy of antithrombin III supplementation in animal models of fulminant Escherichia Coli endotoxemia or bacteremia. Am J Med 87:27 S
19. Triantaphyllopoulos DC (1984) Effect of human antithrombin III on mortality and blood coagulation induced in rabbits by endotoxin. Thromb Haemost 51:232
20. Uchiba M, Okaijma K, Murakami K, Okabe H, Takatsuki K (1996) Attenuation of endotoxin-induced pulmonary vascular injury by antithrombin III. Am J Physiol 270:L921
21. Harada N, Okaijima K, Kushimoto S, Isobe H, Tanaka K (1999) Antithrombin reduces ischemia/reperfusion injury of rat liver by increasing the hepatic level of prostacyclin. Blood 93:157
22. Baggiolini M, Walz A, Kunkel SL (1989) Neutrophil-activating peptide 1/interleukin 8, a novel cytokine that activates neutrophils. J Clin Invest 84:1045
23. Baggiolini M, Clark-Lewis I (1992) Interleukin-8, a chemotactic and inflammatory cytokine. FEBS Lett 307:97
24. Hisama H, Yamaguchi Y, Okaijima K, Uchiba M, Murakami M, Mori K, Yamada S, Ogawa M (1996) Anticoagulant pretreatment attenuates production of cytokine-induced neutrophil chemoattractant following ischemia-reperfusion of rat liver. Dig Dis Sci 41: 1481
25. Jochum M (1995) Influence of high-dose antithrombin concentrate therapy on the release of cellular proteinases, cytokines, and soluble adhesion molecules in acute infalmmation. Semin Hematol 32:19
26. Fourrier F, Chopin C, Huart JJ, Runge I, Caron C, Goudemand J (1993) Double-blind, placebo-controlled trial of antithrombin III concentrates in septic shock with disseminated intravascular coagulation. Chest 104: 882
27. American College of Chest Physiscians/Society of Critical Care Medicine Consensus Conference (1992) Definitions for sepsis and organ failure and guidelines for the use of innovative therapies in sepsis. Crit Care Med 20:864
28. Kurosawa S, Stearns-Kurosawa DJ, Carson CW, D'Angelo A, Della Valle P, Esmon CT (1998) Plasma levels of endothelial cell protein C receptor are elevated in patients with sepsis and systemic lupus erythematosus: lack of correlation with thrombomodulin suggests involvment of different pathological processes. Blood 91:725
29. Beutler B, Cerami A (1987) Cachectin: more than a tumor necrosis factor. New Engl J Med 316:379

30. Tracey KJ, Fong Y, Hesse DG, Manogue KR, Lee AT, Kuo GC, Lowry SF, Cerami A (1987) Anti cachectin/TNF monoclonal antibodies prevent septic shock during lethal bacteraemia. Nature 330:662
31. Waage A, Halstensen A, Espevik T (1987) Association between tumor necrosis factor in serum and fatal outcome in patients with meningococcal disease. Lancet 1:335
32. Oppenheim JJ, Gery L (1982) Interleukin-1 is more than an interleukin. Immunology Today 3:113
33. Bailly S et al.(1994) Comparative production of IL-1βb and IL-1αa by LPS-stimulated human monocytes: ELISAs measurements revisited. Cytokine 6:111
34. Mizel SB (1982) Interleukin-1 and T-cell activation. Immunol Rev 63:51
35. Dinarello CA (1985) An update of human interleukin-1: from molecular biology to clinical relevance. J Clin Immunol 5:287
36. Dinarello CA (1984) Interleukin-1 and the pathogenesis of the acute phase response. N Engl J Med 311:1413
37. Moscovitz H et al.(1994) Plasma cytokine determination in emergency department patients as predictor of bacteremia and infectious disease severity. Crit Care Med 22: 1102
38. Baggiolini M et al.(1989) Neutrophil-activating peptide-1/interleukin-8, a novel cytokine that activates neutrophils. J Clin Invest 84:1045
39. Hack C et al.(1992) Interleukin-8 in sepsis: relation to shock and inflammatory mediators. Infect Immun 60:2835
40. Banchereau J (1990) Interleukin-4. Medecine/Science 6:946
41. Briscoe DM, Cotran RS, Pober JS (1992) Effects of tumor necrosis factor, lipopolysaccharide and IL-4 on the expression of vascular cell adhesion molecules-1 in vivo: correlation with CD3+ T cell infiltration. J Immunol 149:2954
42. Bogdan C, Bodovotz Y, Nathan C (1991) Macrophage deactivation by interleukin-10. J Exp Med 174:1549
43. Marchant A, Deviere J, Byl B, De Groote D, Vincent JL, Goldman M (1994) Interleukin-10 production during septicaemia. Lancet 343:707
44. Lasky LA (1992) Selectins: interpreters of cell-specific carbohydrate information during inflammation. Science 964
45. Cotran RS, Gimbrone MA Jr, Bevilacqua MP, Mendrick DL, Pober JS (1986) Induction and detection of a human endothelial activation antigen in vivo. J Exp Med 164:661
46. Elices MJ, Osborn L, Takada Y, Crouse C, Luhowskyj S, Hemler ME, Lobb RR (1990) VCAM-1 on activated endothelium interacts with the leukocyte integrin VLA-4 at a site distinct from the VLA-fibronectin binding site. Cell 60:577
47. Bevilacqua MP, Stengelin S, Gimbrone MA Jr, Seed B (1989) Endothelial leukocyte adhesion molecule 1: an inducible receptor for neutrophils related to complement regulatory proteins and lectins. Science 243:1160
48. Osborn L, Hession C, Tizard R, Vassalo C, Luhovskyj S, Chi-Rosso G, Lobb RR (1989) Direct expression cloning of vascular cell adhesion molecule 1, a cytokine-induced endothelial protein that binds to lymphocytes. Cell 59:1203
49. Fries JWU, Williams AJ, Atkins RC, Newman W, Lipscomb MF, Collins T (1993) Expression of VCAM-1 and E-selectin in an in vivo model of endothelial activation. Am J Pathol 143:725
50. Fukudome K, Esmon CT (1994) Identification, cloning and regulation of a novel endothelial cell protein C/activated protein C receptor. J Biol Chem 269:26486

51. Regan LM, Stearns-Kurosawa DJ, Kurosawa S, Mollica J, Fukudome K, Esmon CT (1994) The endothelial cell protein C receptor: inhibition of activated protein C anticoagulant function without modulation of reaction with proteinase inhibitors. J Biol Chem 271: 17499
52. Laszik Z, Mitro A, Taylor FB Jr, Ferrel G, Esmon CT (1997) The human protein C receptor is present primarily on endothelium of large blood vessels: implications for the control of the protein C pathway. Circulation 96:3633
53. Stearns-Kurosawa DJ, Kurosawa S, Mollica JS, Ferrell GL, Esmon CT (1996) The endothelial cell protein C receptor augments protein C activation by the thrombin–thrombomodulin complex. Proc Natl Acad Sci USA 93:10212
54. Kurosawa S, Stearns-Kurosawa DJ, Hidari N, Esmon CT (1997) Identification of functional endothelial protein C receptor in human plasma. J Clin Invest 100:411

Treatment of DIC with Antithrombin III in Patients Admitted to Intensive Care Units

F. Baudo, F. de Cataldo, T. M. Caimi, and G. Calori

Introduction

Disseminated intravascular coagulation (DIC) is a syndrome associated with many clinical conditions and may complicate the clinical course and the prognosis of the underlying disease [1, 2]. The clinical picture is characterized by hemorrhagic and/or thrombotic manifestations and sometime by signs and symptoms of organ failure that may complicate the outcome itself [2–4]; the laboratory data are indicative of activation of coagulation and fibrinolytic system and by consumption of the physiological inhibitors (mainly antithrombin III [ATIII]. The clinical conditions frequently associated with DIC are reported in Table 1.

The goal of therapy in DIC is dual: identification of the underlying disorders and the correction of the hemostatic dysfunction with prevention of multi-organ failure. Fresh frozen plasma, specific coagulation factor concentrates, and platelet concentrates have been used to correct the hemostatic defect: the risk of further activation of coagulation with these therapeutic measures was suggested but not unequivocally proved. Similarly, there is no conclusive evidence that

Table 1. Clinical conditions associated with DIC

Obstetric complications: amniotic fluid embolism, placenta abruption, retained fetus syndrome, eclampsia, abortion
Septicemia: Gram negative (endotoxin), Gram positive (mucopolysaccharides)
Neoplastic diseases: metastasis of solid tumors, acute promyelocytic leukemia, acute myelo-monocytic leukemia
Intravascular hemolysis: hemolytic transfusion reactions, acute autoimmune hemolytic anemia, drug related hemolysis
Burns, crush injuries and tissue necrosis, trauma
Acute liver disease
Vascular disorders: giant hemangiona
Metabolic alterations: acidosis

heparin reduces morbidity and mortality. ATIII concentrates are another option for the control of the hemostatic defect and the prevention of the organ dysfunction.

In the intensive care units (ICU), sepsis is one of the most serious complications and a frequent cause of death. The pathology of DIC and the ensuing metabolic changes are very complex and this complexity is the likely cause of the present situation. The mortality of the severe form, in spite of the improvement of anti-microbial therapy and of the supportive procedures in the last 30 years, is still 35%–45% [5–9]; no single therapeutic agent has significantly reduced the overall mortality [10]. DIC in sepsis and septic shock is well documented but only recently we have better understood its pathogenesis and considered new therapy. DIC has an important role in the onset and course of multiple organ dysfunction syndrome (MODS) [11–13]: thrombin is generated with depletion of the coagulation factors and of the physiological inhibitors (mainly ATIII), thrombocytopenia and deposition of fibrin in the microvascular bed [14]. In the early phase of sepsis the fibrinolytic system is activated with generation of plasmin but, as sepsis progresses to severe sepsis and septic shock, it is inhibited by the increased release of the plasminogen activator 1 (PAI 1) induced by tumor necrosis factor (TNF)-α, endotoxin, IL-1, IL-6 and thrombin [15, 16]. In patients with septic shock, a higher lever of PAI 1 was reported [15, 17, 18] and its entity, at the onset of fever in neutropenic patients, predicted a fatal outcome (100% specificity and 92% sensitivity) [19]. The inhibition of fibrinolysis contributes to the persistence of fibrin in the microvascular bed and to the progression to MODS [20]. The role of DIC in sepsis is further suggested by the correlation between the plasma level of ATIII and the outcome.

Functions of ATIII

ATIII is a glycoprotein synthesized in the liver and is the most active physiological inhibitor of the serine proteases generated during blood coagulation (thrombin, factors Xa, IXa, XIa, XIIa), and of kallikrein and plasmin, forming an irreversible complex between the serine residue in the active site of the proteases and an arginine-serine bond in the ATIII [21–23]; its action is increased 1000-fold by heparin and heparan sulfate [24]. Experimental data suggest that ATIII also has anti-inflammatory properties through the release of PGI_2 from the endothelial cells [25–28]. PGI_2 inhibits the activation of the leukocytes and their adhesion to the endothelial cells, and the release of oxygen radicals, lyposomal proteinases and cytokines [29, 30]. ATIII has therefore a vascular protective effect reducing the vascular permeability and the thrombogenicity of the injured wall surfaces [31]. Heparin prevented the release of PGI_2, probably by preventing the interaction of ATIII with the glycosaminoglycans (GAGs) of the endothelial cells [25].

Rationale of ATIII Therapy in Sepsis

Experimental and clinical observations suggest a possible therapeutic role of the ATIII in sepsis: (1) the ATIII plasma concentration is constantly decreased in patients with sepsis or septic shock; (2) the reduction is directly correlated with the severity of the clinical picture; it is a prognostic factor of poor outcome and correlates with survival [15, 32–38]. A significantly lower level of ATIII after surgery was observed in the patients who developed sepsis and in non-survivors [35, 39]. An ATIII concentration above 50% is a favorable prognostic factor for survival (sensitivity of 96% and specificity of 76%) [12]. A value of ATIII below 70% at the onset of fever in patients with leukemia and lymphoma and chemotherapy-related neutropenia is predictive for a lethal outcome (sensitivity and specificity of 85%) [16].

Early clinical studies addressed the use of ATIII in DIC, referring mainly to the modifications of the laboratory parameters. Furthermore, they included a small number of patients with diseases of different etiology and often in very critical conditions. The number of controlled clinical studies is very limited and some of them did not include a placebo group. Normalization of the laboratory data was a common observation but the effect on survival was inconsistent.

In the early 1980s two randomized studies by the same group addressed the use of ATIII concentrates in DIC, in sepsis and shock, but they did not include a placebo arm [37, 40]. Blauhut et al. randomized 51 patients with DIC and shock of different etiology (16 sepsis, 29 trauma, six hepatic coma) to receive ATIII at a dose adjusted to achieve and maintain a normal plasma level, as well as heparin and ATIII + heparin. The main end point was the duration of laboratory data of DIC. The time to response, evaluated by the spontaneous recovery of ATIII activity, and also by the increase of the platelet-count and/or of the fibrinogen concentration, was significantly shorter in the patients receiving ATIII ($p<0.0001$). Twelve deaths were reported without differences in the three groups. A significant decrease of the platelet count and increase of the hemorrhagic complications requiring blood transfusions were recorded when ATIII was combined with heparin ($p<0.03$). In this study only one third of the patients was in shock [40] (Table 2). In a subsequent study, which included only patients with traumatic shock, Vinazzer reported a significant reduction of mortality rate from 31% to 13% in the patients treated with ATIII versus patients treated with heparin alone. This difference was more significant in the subgroup of patients in phase IV shock (defined as coagulation tests with fully developed consumption coagulopathy) [41] (Table 3). In 1995 these data were updated. At this time 170 patients with shock were treated with heparin or ATIII (85 in each group): a significantly better survival was observed in the ATIII-treated group (87% vs 69%; $p<0.005$) [41].

Diaz-Cremades et al. in 1991 designed a prospective, open trial in patients with sepsis and trauma admitted to the intensive care unit (ICU). A total of 36 patients were randomized to receive ATIII or no treatment; 18 of them fulfilled the sepsis criteria. Five patients were in septic shock. No patients had clinically overt DIC. Twenty patients received a standard dose of ATIII (60 U/kg) followed by 10 U/kg every 6 h without dose adjustment. Therapy was discontinued on discharge from the ICU or if ATIII levels remained above 90% for at least 48 h. A better APACHE II score but no difference in survival was observed in the treated group [42]. Balk reported on 34 patients with clinical sepsis: 20 of them were

Table 2. Therapy with ATIII in patients with shock: time to normalization of laboratory data indicative of DIC

Therapy	Dose	Patients number	Diagnosis		Baseline ATIII %	Hours[a]
Heparin	bolus of 3,000 U followed by 250 U/h	17	– sepsis – trauma – hepatic coma	4 11 2	[b]	110
ATIII	dose calculated to obtained ATIII level of 100%	17	– sepsis – trauma – hepatic coma	6 10 1	[b]	42
Heparin ATIII	as above bolus of 1,000 U followed by 100 U/h	17	– sepsis – trauma – hepatic coma	6 8 3	[b]	57
		51			52±9	

[a] Time to normalization of laboratory data indicative of DIC
[b] Not indicated in each group

Table 3. Therapy with ATIII in patients with traumatic shock

	Patients	Mortality (%)	*p*
Shock			
Heparin	85	24 (31)	
ATIII	85	11 (13)	<0.005
Shock phase IV[a]			
Heparin	17	14 (82)	
ATIII	20	6 (30)	<0.001

[a] Decompensated DIC

in shock. A low incidence of laboratory signs consistent with DIC and only slightly reduced mean values of ATIII were present at enrollment in both groups. Eighteen patients received 3000 U of ATIII as bolus followed by 1500 U/day for 5 days; 16 received 2% albumin solution with the same modality. No difference in mortality was observed (12.5% in the placebo vs 22.2% in the ATIII group [43] (Table 4). Fourrier et al. reported the results of a randomized study in 35 patients with septic shock. Here, 17 patients received 5% albumin solution as placebo and 18 patients a dose of ATIII (90–120 U/kg) to obtain and maintain a supranormal level over 5 days. Control of DIC defined as the disappearance of at least one of the laboratory DIC parameters (thrombocytopenia, decrease of

Table 4. Therapy with ATIII in patients admitted to intensive care units: randomized pilot studies

Author	Therapy	Clinical diagnosis	Patients (*n*)	APACHE score (±SD)	ATIII % (±SD)	Mortality (%)
Diaz-Cremades [42]	ATIII	Sepsis	10	16 (4)	52 (11)	35
		Shock	3			
		Trauma	7			
	Non-ATIII	Sepsis	8	15 (5)	48 (12)	31.5
		Shock	2			
		Trauma	6			
Balk [43]	ATIII	Sepsis (Shock)	18 (12)	19 (6)	75 (18)	22
	Placebo	Sepsis (Shock)	16 (10)	17 (7)	78 (10)	12.5

factor V, presence of fibrin monomers) was rapidly achieved in a large number of patients in the ATIII group ($p<0.05$). Survival was not significantly different although there was a trend towards a better outcome in the treated arm (18% reduction of mortality in the intention-to treat analysis, 44% when early deaths were excluded) [44].

Schuster reported the results of a prospective, double-blind, placebo-controlled study in 42 patients with severe sepsis. Twenty patients received placebo and 22 received ATIII (3000 U loading dose, 1500 U twice daily for 5 days). All patients received heparin 6 U/kg per hour through the entire treatment period. The 30-day mortality was not significantly different (41% in the placebo vs 25% in the ATIII group) but again a positive trend in survival and a decreased occurence of multiple organ failure were observed in the treated group [45].

Eisele et al. reported on the results of the North Western European, randomized, double-blind, placebo controlled study carried out in patients with severe sepsis and septic shock. Twenty patients received a loading dose of 3000 U of ATIII, 22 placebo; subsequently ATIII (1500 U) or placebo were infused every 12 h for 5 days. A 39% reduction of mortality was reported in the treated group but the difference was not significant. In the same paper a meta-analysis of the three trials of Fourrier, Eisele and Schuster confirmed the positive trend in the reduction of mortality (45% in the placebo group vs 35% in the treated group) [46]. The low number of the patients enrolled in each study and the addition of heparin in the German study may have confounded the results.

In 1990 we planned a randomized placebo-controlled study to evaluate the effect of the ATIII replacement therapy in a selected group of patients admitted to ICU requiring hemodynamic and/or respiratory support [47]. 120 patients were enrolled, 56 of whom were in septic shock. The patients received a fixed loading dose of 4000 U of ATIII (or 5% albumin solution as placebo) followed by the same dose every 24 h by continuous infusion. Overall survival was not different in the two arms; at day 30, 30 patients in the ATIII group (50%) and 27 patients in the placebo group (46%) were alive. The distribution of the patients was unbalanced because the patients with septic shock and requiring hemodynamic support were more numerous, by chance, in the ATIII treated group (33 versus 23 and 53 versus 42, respectively). The Cox analysis was carried out to determine the net weight of treatment after adjusting for these variables: treatment with ATIII decreases the risk of death with an odds ratio of 0.56. Septic shock was negatively associated with survival; in the post hoc analysis this selected population of patients benefits from ATIII replacement therapy [47].

The limited number of patients enrolled may explain the lack of significant effect on survival in the single studies. A meta-analysis of the three trials, published as full papers, in patients with severe sepsis and/or septic shock was carried out. The analyzed studies are prospective , randomized and the enrolled patients are homogeneous for diagnosis, clinical characteristics, and treatment modality (Tables 5, 6). The end point was mortality at days 28–30. The data were analyzed by META statistical software using the fixed and the random effect models. The studies have not been weighed according to their quality, given the arbitrariness of any weighing procedures. Efficacy results are reported as global odds-ratio (OR) and 95% confidence intervals. Although the ATIII treatment is

Table 5. Characteristics of the patients included in the meta-analysis (septic shock)

Authors	Therapy	Patient (*n*)	Age (years ± SD)	SAP score (± SD)	Baseline ATIII % (± SD)
1. Fourrier [44]	Placebo	18	52 (18)	19 (6)	44 (16)
	ATIII	14	52 (22)	20 (7)	52 (20)
2. Baudo [47]	Placebo	23	63 (8)	18 (6)	46 (16)
	ATIII	33	62 (10)	16 (5)	47 (15)
3. Eisele [46]	Placebo	22	58 (14)	15 (5)[a]	49 (19)
	ATIII	20	57 (16)	13 (5)[a]	46 (14)

[a] APACHE II score

Table 6. Results of the studies included in the meta-analysis: mortality at day 28–30 and surragate "end points"

Authors	Therapy	ATIII[a] (%)	% Mortality (% reduction)	*p*	Surrogate end points[b]	*p*
1. Fourrier [44]	Placebo	<70	50	n.s.	33	<0.05
	ATIII	150–200	28 (↓ 44)		71	
2. Baudo [47]	Placebo	57	87	0.04	8	n.s.
	ATIII	102	30 (↓ 30)		32	
3. Eisele [46]	Placebo	<70	41	n.s.	50	0.09
	ATIII	>70	25 (↓ 39)		16	

[a] Mean ATIII plasma level throughout the treatment period.

[b] Surrogate end points: 1, durations of DIC (% of patients cured at day 4); 2, % variations of MOF score at day 7; 3, length to stay in ICU (% of survivors discharged before day 18)

Table 7. Results of the meta-analysis: effect of ATIII on mortality: global odd ratio (OR) and confidence interval (CI) 95%

Authors	ATIII No. of patients included/dead (%)	Placebo Patients number included/dead (%)	OR	CI 95%	*p*
Fourrier [44]	14/4 (28)	18/9 (50)	0.42	0.10–1.71	
Baudo [47]	33/23 (70)	23/20 (87)	0.39	0.11–1.35	
Eisele [46]	20/5 (25)	22/9 (41)	0.50	0.14–1.77	
Meta-analysis	67/32 (48)	63/38 (60)	0.43	0.20–0.92	0.029

not significantly superior to placebo in the single studies, in the meta-analysis the global OR is statistically significant: 0.43 (CI 0.20–0.92) (Table 7). The lack of statistical significance in each single study could be due to the insufficient number of the patients included [48]. Some questions should be addressed on the clinical use of ATIII concentrate:

1. Who should be treated? The populations in the different trials include a large number of patients with septic shock or severe sepsis; the reduction of death observed in these patients suggests that this particular indication should be investigated.
2. When should treatment be started? In most of the clinical trials the patients were enrolled in critical conditions with established severe sepsis or septic shock and multiple organ failure. Notwithstanding these clinical conditions, a trend of improved survival was reported. Early ATIII treatment is suggested because DIC precedes the development of MODS.
3. What doses should be used? The doses of ATIII used in the different trials is heterogeneous but experimental data and clinical trials stress the importance of using high-doses to maintain a supranormal level of ATIII [30, 49, 50].
4. How long should ATIII be administered? In all the studies the treatment period was limited to 4–5 days and a plateau curve of survival was observed many days after interruption of ATIII therapy. Probably the ATIII was stopped too early before the triggering of DIC had been completely controlled.

The results of each cinical study and of the meta-analysis suggest that a phase III study in patients with severe sepsis and septic shock is opportune.

References

1. Baker WF (1989) Clinical aspects of disseminated intravascular coagulation: a clinician's point of viwe. Semin Thromb Hemost 15:1–57
2. Bick RL (1996) Disseminated intravscular coagulation: objective clinical and laboratory diagnosis, treatment, and assessment of therapeutic response. Semin Thromb Hemost 22:69–88
3. Lerner RG (1976) The defibrination syndrome. Med Clin North Amer 60:871–80
4. Muller-Berghaus G (1977) Pathophysiology of generalized intravascular coagulatio. Semin Thromb Hemost 3:209–246
5. Bone RC, Fisher CJ Jr, Clemmer TP, Slotman GJ, Metz CA, Balk RA (1989) Sepsis syndrome: a valid clinical entity. Crit Care Med 17:389–393
6. Bone RC (1989) Sepsis and coagulation. An important link. Chest 101:594–596
7. Fisher CJ, Dhainaut JFA, Opal SM, Pribble JF, Balk RA, Slothan GJ, Ibertie TJ, Rackow EC, Shapiro MJ, Greenman CL, Reines HD, Shelly MP, Thompson BW, Labrecque SF, Catalano MA, Knaus WA, Sadoff JC (1994) Recombinant human interleukin-1 receptor antagonist in the treatment of patients with sepsis syndrome. JAMA 271:1836–1843
8. Range-Frausto M, Pittet D, Costigan M, Hwang T, Davis CS, Wenzel RP (1995) The natural history of the systemic inflammatory response syndrome (SIRS): a prospective study. JAMA 273:117–123
9. Pinner RV (1996) Trends in infectious disease mortality. JAMA 275:189–192
10. Bernard GR (1995) Sepsis trials, intersection of investigation, regulation, funding, and practice. Am J Resp Crit Care Med 152:4–10
11. Bone RC (1992) Modulators of coagulation: a critical appraisal of their role in sepsis. Arch Intern. Med 152:1381–1389
12. Fourrier F, Chopin C, Goudemand J, Hendrex S, Caron C, Mareu A, Lestavel P (1992) Septic shock, multi organ failure and disseminated intravascular coagulation. Compared pattern of ATIII, protein C, protein S deficiencies. Chest 101:816–823
13. Levi M, ten Cate H, van der Poll T, van Deventer SJH (1993) Pathogenesis of disseminated intravascular coagulation in sepsis. JAMA 270:975–999
14. Vervloet MG, Thijs LG, Hack CE (1998) Derangements of coagulation and fibrinolysis in critically ill patients with sepsis and septic shock. Semin Thromb Hemostas 24:33–44
15. Hesselvik JF, Blombäck M, Brodin B, Maller R (1989) Coagulation, fibrinolysis and kallicrein system in sepsis. Relation to out-come. Crit Care Med 17:724–733
16. Mesters RM, Mannucci PM, Coppola R, Keller T, Ostermann H, Kienast J (1996) Factor VIIa and antithrombin III activity during severe sepsis and septic shock in neutropenic patients. Blood 88:881–886
17. Pralong G, Calandra T, Glauser M-P, Schellekens J, Verhoet S, Bachmann F, Kruithof EK (1989) Plasminogen activator inhibitor I: a new prognostic marker in septic shock. Thromb Haemost 61:459–462
18. Brandtzaeg P, Joo GB, Brusletto B, Kierulf P (1990) Plasminogen activator inhibitor 1 and 2, alpha-2-antiplasmin, plasminogen, and endotoxin levels in systemic meningococcal disease. Thromb Res 57:271–278
19. Mesters RM, Flörke N, Ostermann H, Kienast J (1996) Increase of plasminogen activator inhibitor levels predict outcome of leukocytopenic patients with sepsis. Thromb Hemost 75:902–907

20. Carrico CJ, Meakins JL, Marshall JC, Fry D, Maier RV (1986) Multiple organ failure syndrome. Arch Surg 121:196–208
21. Highsmith RF, Rosenberg RD (1974) The inhibition of human plasmin by human antithombin-heparin cofactor. J Biol Chem 249:4335–4342
22. Bulled HR, Ten Cate JW (1989) Acquired antithrombin III deficiency: laboratory diagnosis, incidence, clinical implications and treatment with antithrombin III concentrate. Am J Med 87(suppl 3B): 44s-48s
23. Rosenberg RD, Bauer KA (1994) The heparin-antithrombin system: a natural anticoagulant mechanism. In: Colman RW, Hirsh J, Marder VJ, Salzman EW, eds. Hemostasis and thrombosis Basic Principles and Clinical Practice. Philadelphia, PA: Lippincott : 837–860
24. Jordan RE, Oosta GM, Gardner WT, Rosenberg RD (1980) The kinetics of hemostatic enzyme-antithrombin interactions in the presence of low molecular weight heparin. J Biol Chem 255:10081–10096
25. Yamanuchi T, Umeda F, Inoguchi I, Nawata H (1989) Antithrombin III stimulates prostacyclin production by cultured aortic endothelial cells. Biochem Biophys Res Commun 163:1404–1411
26. Horie S, Ishii H, Kazama M (1990) Heparin-like glycosaminoglycan is a receptor for antithrombin III-dependent but not for thrombin-dependent prostacyclin production in human endothelial cells. Thromb Res 59:895–904
27. Taylor Jr FB, Chang ACK, Peer GT, Mather T, Blick K, Catlett R, Lockhart MS, Esmon CT (1991) DEGR-factor Xa blocks disseminated intravascular coagulation initiated by Escherichia coli without preventing shock or organ damage. Blood 78:364–368
28. Okijama K, Uchiba M, Murakami K (1998) The anti-inflammatory properties of antithrombin III: new therapeutic implications. Semin Thromb Hemost 24:27–32
29. Jochum, M, Inthorn D, Machleidt W, Waydhas Ch, Friz H (1993) Influence of proteinase inhibitor therapy on the release of cellular proteinase, cytokines and soluble adhesion molecules in acute inflammation. Circ Shock 1:41(a)
30. Jochum M (1995) Influence of high dose antithrombin concentrate therapy on the release of cellular proteinases, cytokines and soluble adhesion molecules in acute inflammation. Semin. Hematol. 32:19–32
31. Uchiba M, Okajima K, Murakami K, Okabe H, Takatsuki K (1996) Attenuation of endotoxin-induced pulmonary vascular injury by antithrombin III. Am J Physiol 270: L921–L930
32. Blauhut B, Necek S, Vinazzer H, Bergmann H (1982) Substitution therapy with an antithrombin III concentrate in shock and DIC. Thromb Res 27:271–278
33. Lammle B, Tran TM, Ritz R, Duckert F (1984) Plasma prekallikrein, factor XII, ATIII, C1-inhibitor and α_2 macroglobulin in critically ill patients with suspected disseminated intravascular coagulation (DIC). Amer J. Clin. Pathol 82:396–404
34. Mammen FE, Hiyakawa T, Phillips TF, Assarian GS, Brown JM, Murano G (1985) Human antithrombin concentrates and experimental disseminated coagulation. Semin Thromb Hemostas 11:373–383
35. Wilson RF, Mammen EF, Robson MC, Heggers JP, Soullier G, DePoli P.A (1986) Antithrombin, prekallikrein and fibronectin levels in surgical patients. Arch Surg 121:635–643
36. Smith-Erichsen N, Aasen AO, Gallimore MJ, Amudsen E (1988) Studies of components of the coagulation system in normal individuals and septic shock patients. Circ Shock 26:227–235

37. Vinazzer H (1989) Therapeutic use of antithrombin III in shock and disseminated intravascular coagulation. Semin Thromb Hemost 15:347–352
38. Sandset PM, Roise O, Aasen AO, Abildgaard U (1989) Extrinsic pathway inhibitor in post operative / post traumatic septicaemia: increased levels in fatal cases. Hemost 19: 189–195
39. Wilson RF, Mammen EP, Tyburski JG, Warsow KM, Kubinec SM (1996) Antithrombin levels related to infections and outcome. J Trauma 40:384–387
40. Blauhut B, Kramar H, Vinazzer H, Bergmann H (1984) Substitution of antithrombin III in shock and DIC: a randomised study. Thromb Res 39:81–89
41. Vinazzer H (1995) Antithrombin III in shock and disseminated intravascular coagulation. Clin Appl Thromb/Hemost 1:62–65
42. Diaz-Cremades JM, Lorenzo R, Sanchez M, Moreno MJ, Alsar MJ, Bosch JM, Fajardo L, Gonzalez D, Guerrero D (1994) Use of antithrombin III in critical patients. Inten Care Med. 20:577–580
43. Balk RA, Bedrosian C, McCormick L, Baughman J, Eisele B, Keinecke HO, Bone RC (1995) Prospective, double-blind, placebo-controlled, trial of ATIII substitution in sepsis. 8th Congress Inten Care Med, Athens S17 (abstr)
44. Fourrier F, Chopin C, Huart JJ, Runge I, Caron C, Goudemand J (1993) Double-blind, placebo-controlled trial of antithrombin III concentrates in septic shock with disseminated intravascular coagulation. Chest 104:882–888
45. Schuster HP, Eisele B, Keinecke HO, Heinrichs H, Mescheder A, Knaub S (1998) S-ATIII study: antithrombin III in patients with sepsis. Inten Care Med 24 (Suppl 1):S76(a)
46. Eisele B, Lamy M, Thijs LG, Keinecke HO, Schuster HP, Matthia FR, Fourrier F, Heinrichs H, Delvos U (1998) Antithrombin III in patients with severe sepsis. A randomized, placebo-controlled, double-blind multicenter trial plus a meta-analysis on all randomized, placebo-controlled, double-blind trials with antithrombin III in severe sepsis. Inten Care Med 24:663–672
47. Baudo F, Caimi TM, deCataldo F, Ravizza A, Arlati S, Casella G, Carugo D, Palareti G, Legnani C, Ridolfi L, Rossi E, D'Angelo A, Crippa L, Giudici D, Gallioli G, Wolfer A, Calori G (1998) Antithrombin III replacement therapy in patients with sepsis and / or post surgical complications: a controlled, double blind, randomized multicenter study. Inten. Care Med. 24:336–342
48. Calori G, Baudo F (1998) Antithrombin III treatment in patients with severe sepsis and septic shock: a meta-analysis. Thromb Res 91 (Suppl 1):S51
49. Kessler CM, Tang ZC, Jacobs HM, Szymanski LM (1997) The suprapharmacologic dosing of antithrombin concentrate for Staphylococcus aureus-induced disseminated intravascular coagulation in guinea pigs: substantial reduction in mortality and morbidity. Blood 89:4393–4401
50. Dickneite G, Paques EP (1993) Reduction of mortality with antithrombin III in septicaemia rats: a study of Klebsiella pneumoniae induced sepsis. Thromb Hemost 69: 98–102

CHAPTER 8

Treatment of Severe Sepsis with C1-Inhibitor

W. A. Wuillemin, S. Zeerleder, C. Caliezi, and C. E. Hack

Introduction

Sepsis has a high mortality rate. Clinical signs and symptoms result from the release and activation of inflammatory mediators. Among these mediators are plasma cascade systems such as the complement systems, the contact activation system and the coagulation system (Fig. 1). Activation of these systems has indeed been demonstrated in sepsis. A typical feature of both the contact and the complement systems is that upon activation they give rise to vasoactive peptides such as bradykinin (contact system) or the anaphylatoxins (complement system). C1-Inhibitor (C1-Inh) is the major inactivator of the component C1 of the complement system and of the contact activation system [60, 69, 74, 84].

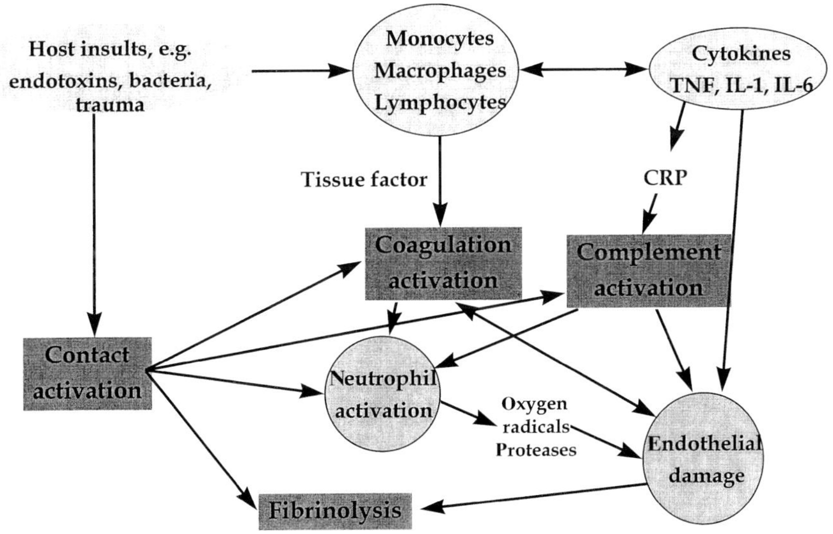

Fig. 1. Activation of host defense systems in sepsis. *CRP*, C-reactive protein; *TNF*, tumor-necrosis factor; *IL*, interleukin

The important physiological role of C1-Inh is best demonstrated by hereditary C1-Inh deficiency and its association with angioedema (HAE) [18, 46]. Attacks of HAE can be effectively treated by intravenous administration of C1-Inh purified from pooled human plasma. Long-term prophylactic substitution with C1-Inh was demonstrated to be safe with hardly any side effects [2, 80].

Because of its inhibitory activity against complement and contact activation, C1-Inh concentrates may be useful for the treatment of diseases other than HAE. Recent studies support this notion. Here we will summarize the biochemistry and biology of C1-Inh. We then will discuss the results of experimental and clinical studies on the therapeutic efficacy of C1-Inh therapy in sepsis.

Biochemistry and Biology of C1-Inh

C1-Inh is a glycosylated single chain polypeptide of 478 amino acid residues, the protein portion of the molecule constituting about 50% of its molecular mass [4]. The molecular weight of C1-Inh is approximately 105 kDa, its plasma concentration around 240 mg/l, or 1 unit (U) per ml [54]. C1-Inh belongs to the superfamily of serine proteinase inhibitors (serpins), which also includes, for example, α1-antitrypsin, antithrombin and plasminogen activator inhibitor type I [7]. Near the carboxy terminal end of the serpin domain is the proteinase recognition region, which is termed the "reactive center loop" [13].

A number of cells, including hepatocytes, fibroblasts, monocytes, macrophages, and endothelial cells are capable of C1-Inh synthesis [3, 43, 44, 78, 85, 87]. Human platelets contain C1-Inh in their α-granules and the platelet levels of C1-Inh correlate with plasma C1-Inh levels [66]. Synthesis of C1-Inh is stimulated by interferon (IFN)-γ and, to a lesser extent, by several other cytokines including tumor necrosis factor-α (TNF-α), IFN-α, monocyte-colony stimulating factor, and interleukin-6 (IL-6) [33, 34, 44, 48, 67, 88]. It was shown that induction of C1-Inh mRNA in IFN-γstimulated cells is primarily due to the enhanced transcription rate of its gene [86]. C1-Inh is therefore an acute phase protein, the plasma levels of which may increase as much as threefold during infections [41].

C1-Inh is encoded by a 17-kb gene on chromosome 11 which consists of eight exons separated by seven introns [9, 15, 72]. The first intron contains IFN-γ-responsive elements that are functional in vitro and that may play a role in IFN-γ-mediated induction of C1-Inh synthesis [87]. The second exon contains the translation initiation site, whereas the DNA encoding the reactive center sequence is situated within exon 8 [17].

Interaction of C1-Inh with target proteinases results in the formation of SDS-stable enzyme–inhibitor complexes and proteolytically cleaved C1-Inh [62]. Analogous to other serpins, C1-Inh inhibits a target proteinase by presenting a peptidyl bond (P1–P1'), lying on an exposed loop within the reactive center that matches the substrate specificity of the proteinase. Attack on this peptidyl bond results in the formation of a complex between inhibitor and proteinase [60, 69, 74]. The complexes formed between C1-Inh and proteinase are removed from the circulation via receptors specific to complexed serpins.

C1-Inh, like most other serpins, can be inactivated by elastase released from activated neutrophils by limited proteolytic cleavage, resulting in the production of socalled "modified C1-Inh" [6, 8, 81]. Likewise, bacterial elastases and proteinases were shown to proteolytically cleave and inactivate C1-Inh [10]. Finally, plasmin was found to play a role in the local cleavage and degradation of C1-Inh in inflammatory processes [79]. The inactivation of C1-Inh may predominantly occur locally in inflamed tissues and, therefore, contribute to increased local complement activation and complement consumption. This conclusion is supported by the demonstration of increased plasma levels of cleaved C1-Inh in patients with sepsis [54].

In normal volunteers the fractional catabolic rate of C1-Inh is 2.5% of the plasma pool per hour, yielding an apparent half-life time of clearance of about 28 h [829. The apparent half-life time of clearance has been reported to be considerably longer in patients with HAE, in whom it may be over 48 h [1, 23].

C1-Inhibitor As Major Inactivator of Several Plasma Cascade Systems

C1-Inh is the only known inhibitor of the activated serine proteinases C1s and C1r from the classical pathway of the complement system, and a major inhibitor of activated factor XII (FXIIa) and kallikrein from the contact activation system, as well as of activated factor XI (FXIa), a proteinase of the intrinsic pathway of the coagulation system. C1-Inh is, therefore, an important regulator of inflammatory reactions and of FXI-dependent clotting activation.

Complement System

The complement system consists of more than 30 serum and cellular proteins, including positive and negative regulators, linked in two biochemical cascades, the classical and alternative pathways (Fig. 2) [50]. The alternative pathway of the complement system is triggered by microbial surfaces and a variety of complex polysaccharides, whereas the classical pathway is usually initiated when a complex of antigen and IgM or IgG antibody binds to the first component of the complement C1. Subsequent activation results in the formation of reactive peptides and the formation of the so-called membrane attack complex, which inserts into target membranes and causes cell lysis [73]. The peptides C3a, C4a, and C5a are known as anaphylatoxins. They mediate several reactions in the inflammatory response, including smooth muscle contractions, changes in vascular permeability, chemotaxis for human mast cells, histamine release from mast cells, and neutrophil chemotaxis as well as platelet activation and aggregation [25, 32, 36].

Activation of the classical pathway of complement is regulated by C1-Inh. It is the only known inhibitor of the activated serine proteinases C1s and C1r [63]. C1-Inh either binds reversibly to proenzymic C1r and C1s within intact C1 to prevent the autoactivation of these proteinases, or binds to activated C1r and C1s and dissociates them from C1q in the form of a C1-Inh–C1r–C1s–C1-Inh tetramer [47]. The rate of inhibition of C1r by C1-Inh is significantly slower than that of C1s.

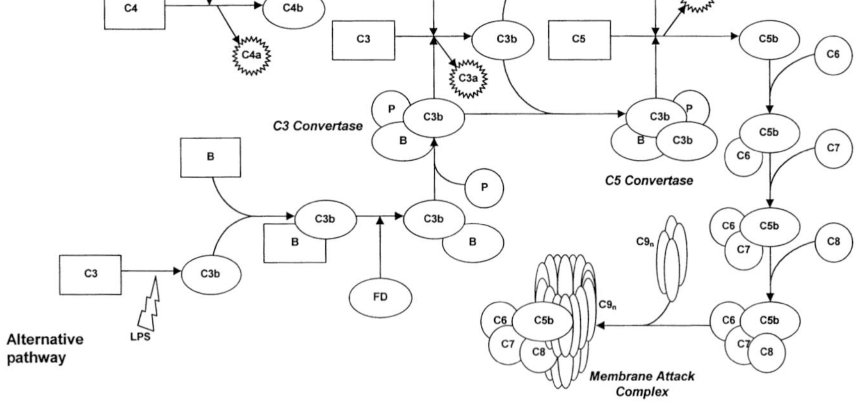

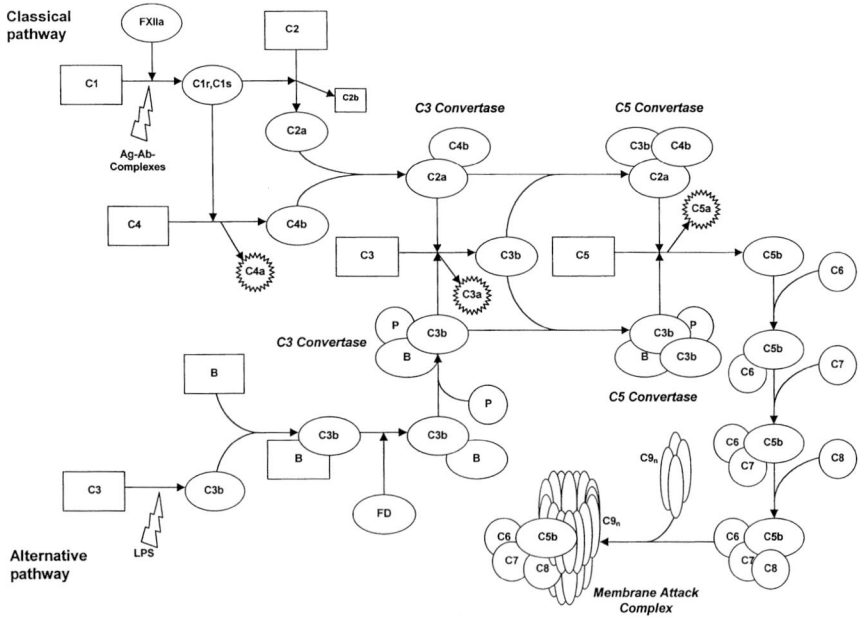

Fig. 2. The complement system. *Ag–Ab complexes*, antigen–antibody-complexes; *LPS*, Lipopolysaccharides; *C*, complement component

Contact Activation System

The proteins factor XII (FXII), prekallikrein (PK), high molecular weight kininogen (HK) and factor XI (FXI) are grouped together as a "contact activation system" (Fig. 3) because they require contact with negatively charged surfaces for zymogen activation [65]. In vitro, FXII and prekallikrein reciprocally activate each other on contact with surfaces and macromolecules such as kaolin, glass, celite, or dextran sulfate. In addition, FXII is able to autoactivate [42].

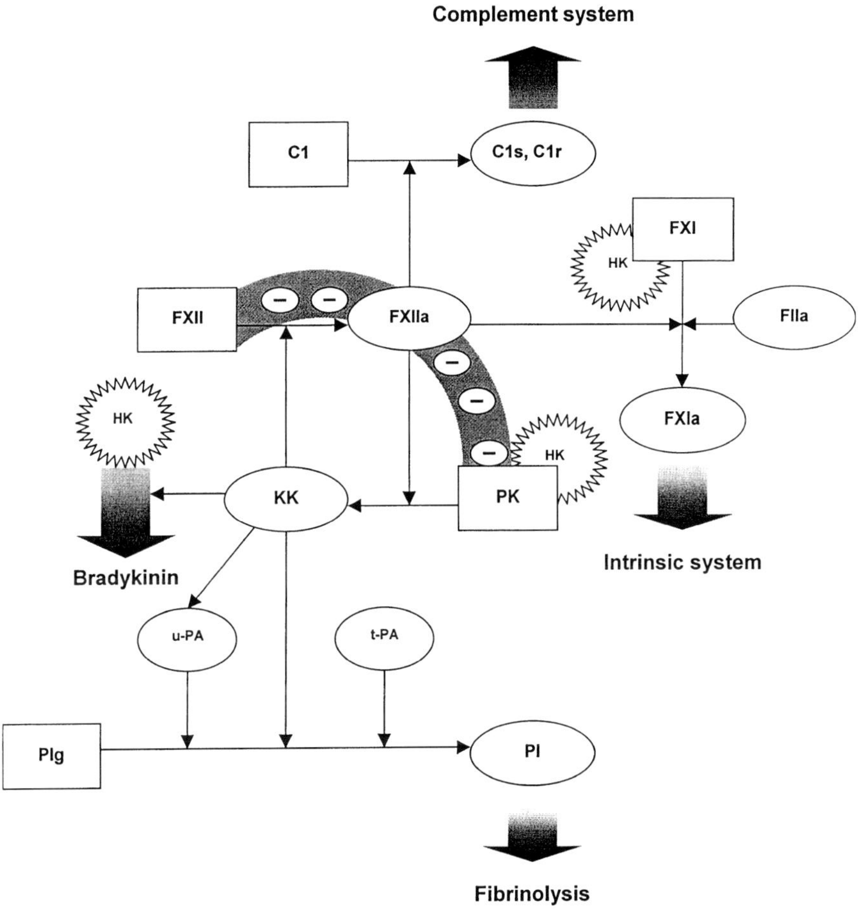

Fig. 3. Contact activation system. *F*, coagulation factor; *a*, activation of the coagulation factor; *C*, complement component; *PK*, prekallikrein; *KK*, kallikrein; *HK*, high molecular weight kininogen; *Plg*, plasminogen; *Pl*, plasmin; *u-PA*, urokinase-type plasminogen activator; *t-PA*, tissue-type plasminogen activator

Cleavage-mediated activation of FXII by kallikrein, FXIa or plasmin leads to the formation of the activated fragments α-FXIIa and β-FXII. The strictly surface-dependent α-FXIIa converts FXI to FXIa, whereas β-FXIIa is an effective prekallikrein activator [42]. Soluble β-FXIIa, but not α-FXIIa, has been shown to activate enzymatically the first component of the complement system by cleavage of the C1r subcomponent [26]. Activated FXII has the ability to cleave plasminogen, rendering it a weak activator of the fibrinolytic system [12]. HK is a nonenzymatic cofactor that augments reciprocal activation of FXII and prekallikrein as well as the rate of FXI activation by FXIIa. HK is the pivotal protein for contact protein assembly on endothelium [65]. Kallikrein activates the fibrinolytic system either by activation of single-chain urokinase or of plasminogen [51]. Finally, kallikrein cleaves HK at two sides to liberate the nonapeptide bradykinin, which is a potent vasoactive peptide [65]. Bradykinin is known to stimulate endothelial cell prostacyclin synthesis, leading to inhibition of platelet function [14], and to increase superoxide formation [35], release of tissue plasminogen activator (t-PA) [70], and nitric oxide formation [57]. In an intact vessel the sum of bradykinin activities is to keep blood flowing and vessels patent. Degradation of bradykinin into inactive fragments depends on the activity of the angiotensin-converting enzyme, which in turn has been documented to be severely decreased in patients with septic shock and septic ARDS [21].

C1-Inh is the major inactivator of α-FXIIa and β-FXIIa and, together with α2-macroglobulin, a major inactivator of kallikrein [60, 62]. Incubation of radiolabelled FXIIa with various plasma proteinases in purified systems and in human plasma demonstrated that FXIIa–C1-Inh complex is the predominant complex to be formed, confirming the major inhibitory role of C1-Inh for FXIIa [60].

Coagulation System

FXI is the coagulation protein that links contact activation to intrinsic blood coagulation. FXI is activated by FXIIa into the active form FXIa by cleavage of an internal peptide bond, giving rise to disulphide linked heavy and light chains [5]. HK serves as a nonenzymatic cofactor in this reaction. Because patients deficient in FXII, prekallikrein, or HK do not suffer from an increased bleeding tendency, contrary to the variable bleeding disorder of patients deficient in FXI, an alternative pathway for the activation of FXI has been assumed and it has been demonstrated that thrombin can activate FXI [24, 52].

Table 1. C1-Inhibitor

Synonyms	C1-esterase inhibitor, C1-inactivator
Classification	Serine proteinase inhibitor (SERPIN)
Abbreviation	C1-Inh
Target proteinases	Complement components C1 s, C1r, coagulation factors α-factor XIIa, β-factor XIIa, kallikrein, factor XIa, and plasmin
Half-life	28–48 h
Concentration	0.24 g/l (range 0.18–3.4)

A current concept of the blood coagulation interactions depicts the tissue factor–FVIIa complex as the initiator of all subsequent reactions: The cell-based TF-FVIIa complex activates both FIX and FX. The FXa-FVa complex then converts prothrombin to thrombin. The amount of thrombin generated in this way is sufficient to activate platelets and activate FV, FVIII and FXI, but it is insufficient for the formation of a stable fibrin clot [61]. Only the subsequent burst of thrombin generation by activated FXI, FIX and FVIII leads to quantitative thrombin generation and the formation of a stable fibrin clot. These data suggest that activation of FXI by thrombin is an alternative pathway for the activation of blood coagulation, and that the role of FXI is to enhance thrombin generation.

Derived from experiments in purified systems, it was suggested that the main inhibitor of FXIa is α1-antitrypsin [68]. However, it could be recently demonstrated in experiments in plasma milieu that C1-Inh is the principle inhibitor of FXIa, followed by α2-antiplasmin, α1-antitrypsin, and antithrombin [84].

Fibrinolytic System

The physiological activators of the fibrinolytic system are tissue-type plasminogen activator (t-PA) and urokinase-like plasminogen activator (u-PA). Both types are serine proteinases that have high activity in converting plasminogen to plasmin [22]. Conversion of the single chain t-PA to the two chain form increases its binding affinity for fibrin [38]. Singlechain u-PA can be rapidly converted to two-chain u-PA by kallikrein and plasmin. Plasma kallikrein has been demonstrated to be a kinetically favorable activator of single-chain u-PA in vitro [39]. Recent studies suggested that the activation of single chain u-PA by kallikrein can best occur on the platelet or endothelial surface [28, 49]. All plasminogen activators share the ability to form plasmin from the inactive zymogen plasminogen. Plasmin is able to hydrolyze fibrinogen, fibrin, FV, FVIII and complement components [22]. In patients with HAE, plasmin–antiplasmin complexes (PAP) were significantly increased during acute attacks, supporting an enhanced activation of the fibrinolytic system via direct activation of plasminogen by kallikrein and FXIIa in a C1-Inh deficiency state [77].

The main inhibitor of single-chain and two-chain t-PA as well as of tow-chain u-PA is plasminogen activator inhibitor type-1 (PAI-1) [45]. The principal physiologic inhibitor of plasmin is α2-antiplasmin. C1-Inh contributes only slowly and to a minor extent to the inactivation of t-PA when t-PA levels are normal [37]. However, when t-PA circulates at high concentrations, e.g., during thrombolytic therapy, or when it is not rapidly cleared from the liver, e.g., in the case of venous occlusion, an increase of circulating t-PA-C1-Inh complexes has been demonstrated [37].

Leukocytes

C1-Inh has been shown to inhibit the activation of CD4+ and CD8+ T-lymphocytes by specific cleavage of the MHC class 1 molecules [19]. In a model of allogen or mitogen-activated murine and human lymphocyte culture systems, the addition of C1-Inh was followed by a downregulation of the activity and proliferation of cytotoxic T-lymphocytes [53]. The addition of C1-Inh altered the production of cytokines by T-lymphocytes, increasing the production of IFN-γ, IL-10 and IL-12 [53].

C1-Inhibitor Therapy in Sepsis and Septic Shock

Sepsis is often induced by bacterial infections and is a leading cause of mortality in noncardiologic intensive care units. Sepsis results from the excessive release and activation of endogenous inflammatory mediators, which include the complement and contact systems. Endothelial injury during the septic process, as suggested by a study with experimentally induced endotoxemia in healthy volunteers [75], or direct activation by bacterial lipopolysaccharides have been proposed as mechanisms leading to activation of the contact factors such as FXII and prekallikrein [11]. Although it has long been supposed that the contact

Table 2. C1-Inh substitution in animal models of sepsis

Condition	Animal	Model	Dosage of C1-Inh	Results	References
Sepsis	Baboons	*E. coli* induced sepsis	500 U/kg bolus i.v. and 200 U/kg over 9 h	Less activation of the contact system (factor XII, prekallikrein) and the complement system (C4b/c)	[40]
Sepsis, hyper-coagulability	Rabbits	*E. coli* endotoxin 120 μg/kg	400 U/kg bolus i.v. and 400 U/kg over 4 h	Stabilization of mean arterial pressure, increase central venous oxygen saturation, reduced fibrin deposition in microcirculation	[64]
Sepsis	Mice deficient in complement C3 and C4	Salmonella typhi endotoxin, 40 mg/kg	200 μg	Less sensitivity to endotoxin, enhanced clearence of endotoxin, improved survival-rate	[20]

system is activated during sepsis, it was not until recently that this concept was proven to be correct: Studies in primates showed decreasing levels of various contact system proteins during sepsis, accompanied by increasing levels of activation products of the contact system [59]. In patients with septic shock, significantly decreased activities of FXII have been demonstrated [41, 55], and in children with meningococcal septic shock, the plasma levels of FXII, FXI and prekallikrein were found to be reduced to about 50% of normal [83]. Definite evidence for the activation of the contact system during the septic process was provided by a study in septic baboons treated before the bacterial challenge with a monoclonal antibody that blocks the activation of FXII [58]. This treatment had no effect on clotting activation but largely prevented irreversible hypotension and slightly improved the survival of baboons challenged intravenously with a lethal dose of *Escherichia coli*. Thus, FXII activation during sepsis does not primarily contribute to clotting derangements, but likely contributes, via the generation of kallikrein and subsequently bradykinin, to the formation of nitric oxide and to vasodilatation [76].

Table 3. C1-inhibitor substitution in patients with sepstic shock

Patients (*n*)	Dosage of C1-Inh	Results	References
5	2000 U followed by 1000 U every 12 h for 5 days	No side effects, less vaso-pressor medication, no death	[31]
6	4000 U followed by two doses of 2000 U and four doses of 1000 U every 12 h or 6000 U followed by 3000 U, 2000 U and 1000 U every 12 h	No side effects, no death	[30]

The role of complement activation during sepsis seems to be dual. Some activation is necessary for an efficient clearance of bacteria or their products. On the other hand, inhibition of the biological effects of C5a in baboons suffering from sepsis attenuated lethal complications [71], illustrating that the pro-inflammatory effects of complement activation, in particular those of C5a, may contribute to the complications of sepsis. Complement component C5a and the membrane attack complex have pro-inflammatory effects such as accumulation and stimulation of neutrophils and may increase the permeability of endothelial cells, mediated in part by histamine, and promote coagulation by inducing expression of tissue factor. The pro-inflammatory effects of complement components during sepsis were supported by observations that C5-deficient mice tolerated endotoxin better than their C5-sufficient littermates [56]. Thus, these studies suggest that during sepsis, complement is required for a rapid clearance of bacteria or their products on the one hand but, on the other hand, via the release of C5a and possibly other fragments, it may enhance inflammatory reactions. Baboons challenged with lethal and sublethal doses of *E. coli* showed a biphasic pattern of complement activation consisting of a rapid initial activation and followed by a second pronounced activation at 24 h [16]. While the initial activation was probably due to a direct stimulation of the complement system, e.g., via IgG or IgM antibodies, the second phase of activation coincided with increasing levels of CRP, IL-2 and IL-6, suggesting a further complement activation via cytokines [16].

Human studies revealed that plasma levels of native complement proteins are decreased in septic patients, while being the lowest in patients with fatal outcome [41]. On the other hand, elevated plasma levels of C3a in patients with sepsis and septic shock were significantly correlated with mortality, and patients with septic shock had significantly higher C3a levels than normotensive patients [29]. The levels of C4a and C1-C1-Inh complexes correlated with C3a levels and with the clinical outcome. It is likely that C5a plays the predominant role in the pathophysiology of the septic processes, because it greatly exceeds C3a in biologic activity; however, measurement of C5a is difficult due to its rapid binding to cellular receptors.

The role of C1-Inh in sepsis was investigated in several clinical studies: In 48 patients with sepsis as compared to healthy volunteers a discrepancy was demonstrated in plasma levels of functional and antigenic C1-Inh that was mainly due to an increase of inactive, cleaved C1-Inh [54]. The extent of plasma C1-Inh proteolysis and the subsequent level of cleaved C1-Inh appeared to be positively correlated with the mortality of the sepsis patients: functional C1-Inh was significantly reduced only in patients with septic shock.

As mentioned above, studies in C4-deficient mice have indicated that an intact classical pathway is required for efficient clearance of endotoxin [20]. Therapeutic C1-Inh administration was demonstrated to incompletely block the activation of the classical pathway and not to interfere with the complement-mediated clearance of bacteria in primates suffering from lethal septic shock [40]. Hence, during C1-Inh administration some opsonization of the infecting microorganisms or their products by the complement system will be preserved.

We have evaluated the effects of therapeutic administration of C1-Inh in a baboon model for lethal *E. coli* septic shock. Administration of C1-Inh at a dose that increased plasma levels 5- to 10-fold reduced activation of C4 and improved mortality [40]. Similarly, a favorable, though mild, effect of C1-Inh has been found in several endotoxin models in rats, dogs, rabbits, and in mice deficient in C4 and C3 [20, 27, 64]. Notably, it has to be established whether the beneficial effects of C1-Inh in sepsis are due to its effect on complement, on the contact system, or on both.

Preliminary evaluation of C1-Inh therapy in patients with septic shock has been performed [30, 31]. Initially, five patients treated with mechanical ventilatory support, volume substitution, vasopressor and positive inotropic drugs received C1-Inh for 5 days, starting with a dose of 2000 U, subsequently followed by 1000 U every 12 h. No patient died during the study period of 5 days. Four of the patients needed less and one patient needed more vasopressor therapy during this period. No side effects of C1-Inh treatment were observed. Both complement and contact system parameters were measured in the five patients who received C1-Inh. C3a levels tended to decrease in these patients [30], whereas FXII levels increased [31]. We then administered C1-Inh to seven additional patients with septic shock, one of whom did not complete the study because of transfer to another hospital. Three patients received C1-Inh for 3 days, a starting dose of 4000 U followed by two doses of 2000 U and four doses of 1000 U every 12 h; the other three patients received 6000 U of C1-Inh followed by 3000, 2000 and 1000 U (all doses given at 12-h intervals). Effects comparable with those of the other dose regimen were seen: no toxic side effects and a slight reduction of complement and contact activation. These results with no toxic side effects, no sepsis-related mortality during the study period, a possible attenuation of complement and contact activation, and a possible beneficial effect on hypotension as reflected by a decreased need for vasopressor medication were confirmed in several open, uncontrolled studies in a limited number of septic shock patients, who all received C1-Inh according to the schemes outlined above (2nd workshop on C1-inhibitor, Düsseldorf, 1997). Therefore, double-blind, controlled studies in a larger number of patients are warranted to confirm these promising effects. Such a study will be completed in 1999 at the University hospital of Berne.

Acknowledgements. WAW and SZ are supported by a grant from the Swiss National Foundation for Scientific Research (Nr. 3200–055312.98).

References

1. Agostoni A, Bergamaschini L, Martignoni G, Cicardi M, Marasini B (1980) Treatment of acute attacks of hereditary angioedema with C1-inhibitor concentrate. Ann Allergy 44:299–301
2. Agostoni A, Cicardi M (1992) Hereditary and acquired C1-inhibitor deficiency: biological and clinical characteristics in 235 patients. Medicine 71:206–215
3. Bensa JC, Reboul A, Colomb MG (1983) Biosynthesis in vitro of complement subcomponents C1q, C1 s and C1 inhibitor by resting and stimulated human monocytes. Biochem J 216:385–392
4. Bock SC, Skriver K, Nielsen E et al (1986) Human C1 inhibitor: primary structure, cDNA cloning, and chromosomal localization. Biochemistry 25:4292–4301
5. Bouma BN, Griffin JH (1977) Human blood coagulation factor XI. Purification, properties and mechanism of activation by activated factor XII. J Biol Chem 252:6432
6. Brower MS, Harpel PS (1982) Proteolytic cleavage and inactivation of α_2-plasmin inhibitor and C1 inactivator by human polymorphonuclear leukozyte elastase. J. Biol Chem 257:9849–9854
7. Carrell RW, Boswell DR (1990) Serpins: the superfamily of plasma proteinase inhibitors. In: Barrett AJ, Salvesen G (eds) Proteinase inhibitors. Elsevier, Amsterdam, pp 403–420
8. Carrell RW, Christey PB, Boswell DR (1987) Serpins: antithrombin and other inhibitors of coagulation and fibrinolysis. Evidence from amino acid sequences. In: Verstraete M, Vermylen J, Lijnen R, Arnout J (eds) Thrombosis and haemostasis. Leuven University Press, Leuven, pp 1–15

9. Carter P, Duponchel C, Tosi M, Fothergill J (1991) Complete nucleotide sequence of the gene of human C1 inhibitor with an unusually high density of Alu elements. Eur J Biochem 197:301–308
10. Catanese J, Kress LF (1984) Enzymatic inactivation of human plasma C1-inhibitor and α_1-antichymotrypsin by *Pseudomonas aeruginosa* proteinase and elastase. Biochim Biophys Acta 789:37–43
11. Colman RW (1994) Disseminated intravascular coagulation due to sepsis. Semin Hematol 31:10–17
12. Colman RW, Bagdasarian A, Talamo RC et al (1975) Williams trait. Human kininogen deficiency with diminished levels of plasminogen proactivator and prekallikrein associated with abnormalities of the Hageman factor-dependent pathway. J Clin Invest 56:1650–1662
13. Coutinho M, Aulak KS, Davis III AE (1994) Functional analysis of the serpin domain of C1 inhibitor. J Immunol 153:3648–3654
14. Crutchley DJ, Ryan JW, Ryan US, Fisher GH (1983) Bradykinin-induced release of prostacyclin and thromboxanes from bovine pulmonary artery endothelial cells. Studies with lower homologs and calcium antagonists. Biochem Biophys Acta 751:99–107
15. Davis III AE, Whitehead AS, Harrison RA et al (1986) Human inhibitor of the first component of complement, C1: characterization of cDNA clones and localization of the gene to chromosome 11. Proc Natl Acad Sci USA 83:3161–3165
16. De Boer JP, Creasey AA, Chang A et al (1993) Activation of the complement system in baboons challenged with live *Escherichia coli*: correlation with mortality and evidence for a biphasic activation pattern. Infect Immun 61:4293–4301
17. Donaldson VH, Bissler JJ (1992) C1-inhibitors and their genes: an update. J Lab Clin Med 119:330–333
18. Donaldson VH, Evans RR (1963) A biochemical abnormality in hereditary angioneurotic edema. Am J Med 35:37–44
19. Eriksson H, Sjögren HO (1995) Inhibition of activation of human T lymphocytes by the complement C1 esterase inhibitor. Immunology 86:304–10
20. Fischer MB, Prodeus AP, Nicholson-Weller A et al (1997) Increased susceptibility to endotoxin shock in complement C3- and C4- deficient mice is corrected by C1 inhibitor replacement. J Immunol 159:976–982
21. Fourrier F, Chopin C, Wallaert B, Mazurier C, Mangalaboyi J, Durocher A. (1985) Compared evolution of plasma fibronectin and angiotensin converting enzyme levels in septic ARDS. Chest 87:191–5
22. Francis CW, Marder VJ (1987) Physiologic regulation and pathologic disorders of fibrinolysis. Hum Pathol 18:263–274
23. Gadek JE, Hosea SW, Gelfand JA et al (1980) Replacement therapy in hereditary angioedema. Successful treatment of acute episodes of angioedema with partly purified C1 inhibitor. N Engl J Med 302:542–546
24. Gailani D, Broze GJJ (1991) Factor XI activation of coagulation in a revisited model of blood coagulation. Science 253:909–912
25. Gerard C, Gerard NP (1994) C5a anaphylatoxin and its seven transmembranesegment receptor. Annu Rev Immunol 12:775–808
26. Ghebrehiwet B, Randazzo BP, Dunn JT, Silverberg M, Kaplan AP (1983) Mechanisms of activation of the classical pathway of complement by Hageman factor fragment. J Clin Invest 71(5):1450–1456
27. Guerrero R, Velasco F, Rodriguez M et al (1993) Endotoxin-induced pulmonary dysfunction is prevented by C1-esterase inhibitor. J Clin Invest 91:2754–2760

28. Gurewich V, Johnstone M, Loza JP, Pannell R (1993) Pro-urokinase and prekallikrein are both associated with platelets. Implications for the intrinsic pathway of fibrinolysis and for thrombotic thrombolysis. FEBS Lett 318:317–321
29. Hack CE, Nuijens JH, Felt-Bersma RJ et al (1989) Elevated plasma levels of the anaphylatoxins C3a and C4a are associated with a fatal outcome in sepsis. Am J Med 86:20–26
30. Hack CE, Ogilvie AC, Eisele B, Erenberg AM, Wagstaff J, Thijs LG (1993) C1 inhibitor substitution therapy in septic shock and in vascular leak syndrome induced by high doses of interleukin-2. Int Care Med 19:19–28
31. Hack CE, Voerman HJ, Eisele B et al (1992) C1 esterase inhibitor substitution in sepsis. Lancet 339:378
32. Hartmann K, Henz BM, Krüger-Krasagakes S et al (1997) C3a and C5a stimulate chemotaxis of human mast cells. Blood 89:2863–2870
33. Heda GD, Kehoe KJ, Mahdi F, Schmaier AH (1996) Phosphatase 2 A participates in Interferon-γ's induced upregulation of C1 inhibitor mRNA expression. Blood 87: 2831–2838
34. Heda GD, Mardente S, Weiner L, Schmaier AH (1990) Interferon γ increases in vitro and in vivo expression of C1 inhibitor. Blood 75:2401–2407
35. Holland JA, Pritchard KA, Papolla MA, Wolin MS, Rogers NJ, Stemerman MB (1990) Bradykinin induces superoxide anion release from human endothelial cells. J Cell Physiol 143:21–25
36. Hugli TE, Müller-Eberhard HJ (1978) Anaphylatoxins: C3a and C5a. Adv Immunol 26: 1–53
37. Huisman LGM, van Griensven JMT, Kluft C (1995) On the role of C1-inhibitor as inhibitor of tissue-type plasminogen activator in human plasma. Thromb Haemost 73: 466–471
38. Husain SS, Hasan AAK, Budzinsky AZ (1989) Differences between binding of one-chain and two-chain tissue plasminogen activators to non-cross-linked and cross-linked clots. Blood 74:999
39. Ichinose A, Fujikawa K, Suyama T (1986) The activation of prourokinase by plasma kallikrein and its inactivation by thrombin. J Biol Chem 261:3486–3489
40. Jansen PW, Eisele B, De Jong IW et al (1998) Effect of C1 inhibitor on inflammatory and physiologic response patterns in primates suffering from lethal septic shock. J Immunol 160:475–484
41. Kalter ES, Daha MR, ten Cate JW, Verhoef J, Bouma BN (1985) Activation and inhibition of Hageman factor-dependent pathways and the complement system in uncomplicated bacteremia or bacterial shock. J Infect Dis 151:1019–1027
42. Kaplan AP, Silverberg M (1987) The coagulation-kinin pathway of human plasma. Blood 70:1–15
43. Katz Y, Gur S, Aladjem M, Strunk RC (1995) Synthesis of complement proteins in amnion. J Clin Endocrinol Metab 80:2027–2032
44. Katz Y, Strunk R (1989) Synthesis and regulation of C1 inhibitor in human skin fibroblasts. J Immunol 142:2041–2045
45. Kruithof EKO, Tran-Thang CH, Bachmann F (1986) The fast-acting inhibitor of tissue-type plasminogen activator in plasma is also the primary plasma inhibitor of urokinase. Thromb Haemost 55:65
46. Landermann NS, Webster ME, Becker EL, Ratcliffe HE (1962) Hereditary angioneurotic edema. II. Deficiency of inhibitor for serum globulin permeability factor and/or plasma kallikrein. Allergy 33:330–341

47. Liszewski MK, Farries TC, Lublin DM, Rooney IA, Atkinson JP (1996) Control of the complement system. Adv Immunol 61:201–283
48. Lotz M, Zuraw BL (1987) Interferon-gamma is a major regulator of C1-inhibitor synthesis by human blood monocytes. J Immunol 139:3382–3387
49. Loza JP, Gurewich V, Johnstone M, Pannell R (1994) Platelet-bound prekallikrein promotes pro-urokinase-induced clot lysis: a mechanism for targeting the factor XII dependent intrinsic pathway of fibrinolysis. Thromb Haemost 71:347–352
50. Makkrides SC (1998) Therapeutic inhibition of the complement system. Pharmacol Rev 50:59–87
51. Motta G, Rojkjaer R, Hasan AAK, Cines DB, Schmaier AH (1998) High molecular weight kininogen regulates prekallikrein assembly and activation on endothelial cells: a novel mechanism for contact activation. Blood 91:516–528
52. Naito K, Fujikawa K (1991) Activation of human blood coagulation factor XI independent of factor XII. Factor XI is activated by thrombin in the presence of negatively charged surfaces. J Biol Chem 266:7353–7358
53. Nissen MH, Bregenholt S, Nording JA, Cleasson MH (1998) C1-esterase inhibitor blocks T lymphocyte proliferation and cytotoxic T lymphocyte generation in vitro. Int Immunol 10:167–173
54. Nuijens JH, Erenberg-Belmer AM, Huijbregts CC et al (1989) Proteolytic inactivation of plasma C1 inhibitor in sepsis. J Clin Invest 84:443–450
55. Nuijens JH, Huijbregts CC, Erenberg-Belmer AM et al (1988) Quantification of plasma factor XIIa-C1-inhibitor and kallikrein-C1-inhibitor complexes in sepsis. Blood 72:1841–1848
56. Olson LM, Moss GS, Baukus O, Das Gupta TK (1985) The role of C5 in septic lung injury. Ann Surg 202:771–776
57. Palmer RMJ, Ferrige AG, Moncada S (1987) Nitric oxide release accounts for the biologic activity of endothelium derived relaxing factor. Nature 327:524–526
58. Pixley RA, De la Cadena R, Page JD et al (1993) The contact system contributes to hypotension but not disseminated intravascular coagulation in lethal bacteremia. J Clin Invest 91:61–68
59. Pixley RA, De la Cadena RA, Page JD et al (1992) Activation of the contact system in lethal hypotensive bacteremia in a baboon model. Am J Pathol 140:897–906
60. Pixley RA, Schapira M, Colman RW (1985) The regulation of human factor XIIa by plasma proteinase inhibitors. J. Biol Chem 260:1723–1729
61. Roberts HR, Monroe DM, Oliver JA, Chang J-Y, Hoffmann M (1998) Newer concepts of blood coagulation. Haemophilia 4:331–334
62. Schapira M, De Agostini A, Colman RW (1988) C1 inhibitor: the predominant inhibitor of plasma kallikrein. Methods Enzymol 163:179–185
63. Schapira M, de Agostini A, Schifferli JA, Colman RW (1985) Biochemistry and pathophysiology of human C1 inhibitor: Current issues. Complement 2:111–126
64. Scherer RU, Giebler RM, Schmidt U, Paar D, Kox WJ (1996) The influence of C1 esterase inhibitor substitution on coagulation and cardiorespiratory parameters in an endotoxin induced rabbit model of hypercoagulability. Sem Thromb Haemost 22:357–366
65. Schmaier AH (1997) Contact activation: A revision. Thromb Haemost 78:101–107
66. Schmaier AH, Amenta S, Xiong T, Heda GD, Gewirtz AM (1993) Expression of platelet C1 inhibitor. Blood 82:465–474
67. Schmidt B, Gyapay G, Valay M, Fust G (1991) Human recombinant macrophage colony-stimulating factor (M-CSF) increases C1-esterase inhibitor (C1INH) synthesis by human monocytes. Immunology 74:677–679

68. Scott CF, Schapira M, James HL, Cohen AB, Colman RW (1982) Inactivation of factor XIa by plasma protease inhibitors. Predominant role of α1-proteinase inhibitor and protective effect of high molecular wight kininogen. J Clin Invest 69:844–852
69. Sim RB, Reboul A, Arlaud GJ, Villiers CL, Colomb MG (1979) Interaction of 125-labelled complement components C1r and C1s with protease inhibitors in plasma. FEBS Lett 97:111–115
70. Smith D, Gilbert M, Owen WG (1983) Tissue plasminogen activator release in vivo in response to vasoactive agents. Blood 66:835–839
71. Stevens JH, O'Hanley P, Shapiro JM et al (1986) Effects of anti-C5a antibodies on the adult respiratory distress syndrome in septic primates. J Clin Invest 77:1818–1826
72. Theriault A, Whaley K, McPhaden A, Boyd E, Connor J (1989) Regional assignment of the human C1 inhibitor gene to 11q11-q13.1. Hum Genet 84:477–479
73. Tschopp J, Müller-Eberhard HJ, Podack ER (1982) Formation of transmembrane tubules by spontaneous polymerization of the hydrophilic complement protein C9. Nature 298:534–538
74. Van den Graaf F, Koedam JA, Bouma BN (1983) Inactivation of Kallikrein in human plasma. J Clin Invest 71:149–158
75. Van Deventer SJH, Büller HR, ten Cate JW, Aarden LA, Hack CE, Sturk A (1990) Experimental endotoxemia in humans: analysis of cytokine release and coagulation, fibrinoltyic, and complement pathways. Blood 76:2520–2526
76. Vane JR, AnggArd EE, Botting RM (1990) Regulatory functions of the vascular endothelium. N Engl J Med 323:27–36
77. Waage Nielsen E, Thidemann Johansen H, Hogasen K, Wuillemin WA, Hack CE, Mollnes TE (1996) Activation of the complement, coagulation, fibrinoltyic and kallikrein-kinin systems during attacks of hereditary angioedema. Scand J Immunol 44:185–192
78. Walker DG, Yasuhara O, Patston PA, McGeer EG, McGeer PL (1995) Complement C1 inhibitor is produced by brain tissue and is cleaved in Alzheimer disease. Brain Res 675: 75–82
79. Wallace EM, Perkins SJ, Sim RB, Willis AC, Feighery C, Jackson J (1997) Degradation of C1-inhibitor by plasmin: Implications for the control of inflammatory process. Mol Med 3:385–396
80. Waytes AT, Rosen FS, Frank MM (1996) Treatment of hereditary angioedema with a vapor-heated C1 inhibitor concentrate. N Engl J Med 334:1630–1634
81. Weiss SJ (1989) Tissue destruction by neutrophils. *N* Engl J Med 320:365–376
82. Woo P, Lachmann PJL, Harrison RA, Amos N (1985) Simultaneous turnover of normal and dysfunctional C1 inhibitor as a probe of in vivo activation of C1 and contact activatable proteases. Clin Exp Immunol 61:1–8
83. Wuillemin WA, Fijnvandraat K, Derkx BH et al (1995) Activation of the intrinsic pathway of coagulation in children with meningococcal septic shock. Thromb Haemost 74: 1436–1441
84. Wuillemin WA, Minnema M, Meijers JC et al (1995) Inactivation of factor XIa in human plasma assessed by measuring factor XIa-protease inhibitor complexes: major role of C1-inhibitor. Blood 85:1517–1526
85. Yeung LA, Jones L, Hamilton AO, Whaley K (1985) Complement-subcomponent-C1-inhibitor synthesis by human monocytes. Biochem J 226:199–205
86. Zahedi K, Prada A, Davis III AE (1994) Transcriptional regulation of the C1 inhibitor gene by γ interferon. J Biol Chem 269:9669–9674

87. Zahedi K, Prada AE, Davis III AE (1997) Characterization of the IFN-γ-responsive element in the 5' flanking region of the C1 inhibitor gene. J Immunol 159:6091–6096
88. Zuraw B, Lotz M (1990) Regulation of the hepatic synthesis of C1 inhibitor by the hepatocyte stimulating factors interleukin 6 and interferon gamma. J Biol Chem 265: 12664–12770

Behandlung der Gefäßdysfunktion im Rahmen einer Sepsis und eines septischen Schocks

F. Schneider, J. C. Stoclet, R. Janssen und J. D. Tempé

Das Eindringen eines infektiösen Agens in den Organismus ruft in diesem komplexe Abwehrmechanismen hervor, die vom Immunsystem gesteuert werden. Die Aufgabe dieser Reaktionen ist die Eliminierung des Antigens und die Begrenzung des schädigenden Einflusses auf den Organismus, mit dem Ziel, seine Unversehrtheit und damit das Leben aufrechtzuerhalten. Die kardiovaskulären Veränderungen, sei es im Rahmen einer einfachen Bakteriämie, einer Endotoxinämie, einer Sepsis oder eines septischen Schocks, unterscheiden sich nicht wesentlich in ihrer Reaktionsart, sondern vielmehr in der Intensität dieser Reaktionen. Das Ausmaß dieser Mechanismen ist individuell nicht vorhersehbar, nimmt aber vor allem bei den klinischen Formen mit Kreislaufkollaps einen wichtigen vitalprognostischen Stellenwert ein.

Da die Behandlung der kardialen Komplikationen anderweitig behandelt wird, werden wir uns hier vorrangig mit den Gefäßveränderungen beschäftigen. Diese Trennung kann jedoch nur artifiziell bleiben, wenn man ihre vielfältigen physiologischen Wechselwirkungen betrachtet. Bevor nun die Behandlungsmöglichkeiten, ihre Indikationsstellung und ihr Wirkungserfolg vorgestellt werden, möchten wir uns die ihnen zugrunde liegenden, physiopathologischen Zusammenhänge ins Gedächtnis rufen.

Pathophysiologie der Gefäßveränderungen bei schwerer Infektion

Der menschliche Organismus reagiert sehr empfindlich auf eindringende körperfremde Antigene, wie zum Beispiel bakterielle Lipopolysaccharide (LPS). Diese provozieren auf der einen Seite Allgemeinsymptome wie Fieber und Unwohlsein und auf der anderen Seite vaskuläre Sofortreaktionen (in der ersten Stunde) und Spätreaktionen (nach vier bis fünf Stunden) [1]; letztere können entweder reversibel sein oder in Form eines hyperkinetischen Schocks mit erhöhtem Herzzeitvolumen und erniedrigtem peripherem Gefäßwiderstand fortbestehen, um dann nach unvorhersehbarer Dauer zum Kreislaufkollaps mit stark erniedrigtem Herzzeitvolumen und erhöhtem peripherem Gefäßwiderstand zu führen [2]. Nicht selten kann man auch Patienten beobachten, die bei vermindertem Herzzeitvolumen nicht mehr in der Lage sind, ihren peripheren Gefäßwiderstand zu erhöhen [3]. In der Intensivmedizin ist die erhöhte Mortalität im Verlauf schwerer Infektionen oft auf die Kreislaufkomplikationen zurückzuführen. Zum heutigen Zeitpunkt existiert keine allgemein anerkannte Antwort auf die Frage, warum ein Patient vom Stadium der einfachen Sepsis mit günstiger Spontanentwicklung in das Stadium eines tödlichen septischen Schocks eintritt.Auf jeden Fall scheint es offensichtlich, daß hierbei unterschiedliche Faktoren zusammenspielen, wie die Virulenz des Antigens und der Zustand des Immunsystems. Angeborene oder erworbene Immundefekte sind in der Tat Faktoren, die das Mortalitätsrisiko erhöhen. Das im Rahmen septischer Erkrankungen beobachtete Kreislaufversagen zeigt, beim Tier wie beim Menschen, eine in Phasen ablaufende Entwicklung [2–5]:

- eine ***Initialphase*** der Gefäßdilatation mit rasch einsetzendem Blutdruckabfall, der normalerweise gut auf verschiedene pharmakologische Substanzen anspricht (meist Agonisten der Vasokonstriktion);
- eine ***Zweitphase***, die nach drei bis vier Stunden einsetzt und einer Phase der Blutdruckinstabilität entspricht, in der die vasodilatatorischen Mechanismen an der Gefäßwand überwiegen und die Anwendung vielfältiger hämodynamisch wirksamer Substanzen erforderlich wird. Der bedeutende interstitielle Flüssigkeitsverlust („leak syndrome") und die dadurch provozierte Hypovolämie erfordern dann eine angemessene Volumensubstitution;
- eine ***dritte Phase***, normalerweise Stunden bis Tage später einsetzend, bei der man entweder eine kontinuierliche Verbesserung der Kreislaufsituation oder im Gegenteil, eine Resistenz gegen jede gefäßaktive Therapie beobachtet, die folglich zum Tod durch Multiorganversagen führt.

Welches sind die verantwortlichen Faktoren der Gefäßveränderungen nach Eindringen des infektiösen Agens?

Bis Mitte der siebziger Jahre war allgemein anerkannt, daß der Wirkungsverlust der Katecholamine in ihrer Funktion der Aufrechterhaltung des Blutdrucks der Grund für die dem septischen Schock zugrunde liegende Gefäßdysfunktionen sei. Folglich wurde der zu niedrige Blutdruck als Ursache für eine unzureichende Organdurchblutung und eine verminderte Sauerstoffversorgung des Gewebes für jene Stoffwechselvorgänge verantwortlich gemacht, die zunächst zur lokalen und schließlich zur systemischen Azidose führten. Man nahm also an, daß diese Mechanismen entweder auf einer Verminderung der Katecholaminproduktion, auf einer herabgesetzten Wirkung auf die Katecholamin-Rezeptoren oder schließlich auf eine Veränderung der Anzahl beziehungweise der Beschaffenheit dieser Rezeptoren zurückzuführen sei [6]. Seit der Endeckung von gewissen Prostaglandinen und ihren Abkömmlingen ist man auf die Idee gekommen, daß vasoaktive Substanzen in der Gefäßwand selbst synthetisiert werden, um hier zunächst lokale vasoregulatorische Funktionen zu übernehmen und letztendlich die systemische Hämodynamik zu beeinflussen [7]. In der Tat hat man in bestimmten Tierversuchsreihen zeigen können, daß der Blutdruckabfall nach Injektion von LPS „in vivo" von einer erhöhten Plasmakonzentration der Eikosanoide begleitet war und daß die Hemmung der Zyklooxygenase zur teilweisen Blutdruckerhöhung bei gewissen experimentellen Infektionen geführt hat [8, 9]. Bisher hat jedoch keine Studie das Zutreffen dieser Hypothese beim Menschen beweisen können.

Während der achtziger Jahre haben hauptsächlich zwei Erkenntnisse unser Wissen über die generalisierte Infektion verändert: zuerst die Entdeckung der Zytokinsynthese als wesentlicher Bestandteil der Immunreaktion im Rahmen einer schweren Infektion [10] und schließlich die Aufklärung der Funktion des Gefäßendothels in der Pathophysiologie der Kreislaufstörungen, die sowohl vom infektiösen Agens als auch von den Zytokinen ausgelöst werden [11]. Somit ist offensichtlich, daß die Zytokine, wie TNF und andere Interleukine, die normalerweise von Zellen des Abwehrsystems produziert werden, in der Lage sind, einen hyperkinetischen Schock hervorzurufen, wenn sie einem Tier oder dem Menschen injiziert werden [12]. Ebenso führt eine schwere Infektion beim Menschen zur Produktion von Zytokinen durch das Abwehrsystem [10]. Man kann also sagen, daß dieses Phänomen für das Auftreten eines hyperkinetisches Syndroms verantwortlich ist.

Ohne den schützenden oder schädigenden Effekt der Zytokin-Synthese zu bewerten, kann man also annehmen, daß im Laufe einer Infektion das Eindringen von Antigenen in den menschlichen Organismus in diesem eine hämodynamische Reaktion auslöst, die einerseits durch die Antigenstrukturen selbst und andererseits durch die Zytokine vermittelt werden.

Welches sind die biologischen Veränderungen der Gefäßphysiologie, die das Überwiegen der Gefäßdilatation im Verlauf einer Sepsis erklären?

Im physiologischen Zustand erlaubt ein feines Gleichgewicht von vasodilatatorischen und vasokonstriktorischen Faktoren eine ausreichende Gewebesauerstoffsättigung. Die Anwesenheit zirkulierender Antigene wird von den Oberflächenrezeptoren der Endothelzellen erkannt [13] und als Information über verschiedene biologische Vermittlungssysteme ins Zytoplasma weitergeleitet. Einer dieser Botenstoffe stellt NF-κB im Zytoplasma dar [14], das sich normalerweise unter dem Einfluß physiologischer Hemmstoffe im Ruhezustand befindet. Im Falle einer Sepsis nimmt es an der Synthesesteigerung von messenger-RNA für gewisse Enzymproteine teil. Zusätzlich zu diesem Botenmechanismus haben die freigesetzten Zytokine selbst die Fähigkeit, die genetische Produktion dieser Proteine auszulösen und somit auch in Abwesenheit des NF-κB die Möglichkeit, den Endothelzellen und auch den glatten Muskelzellen der Gefäßwand die Existenz einer akuten Infektion mitzuteilen: Daraus folgt die Stimulierung der Zellkernaktivität und somit der Proteinbiosynthese. Das Endresultat besteht in der Erhöhung der Konzentration induzierter Enzyme im Zytoplasma des Endothels und der glatten Muskulatur, wie der induzierbaren NO-Synthase (iNOS) [15], der induzierbaren Hämoxygenase [16] und anderer noch nicht genau identifizierter Enzymsysteme. Im Tierversuch ist auch gezeigt worden, daß die Zellreaktion im Falle einer Sepsis eine Erhöhung des intrazellulären Kalziumspiegels zur Folge hat [17] – ein notwendiges Phänomen für die Funktionsfähigkeit gewisser Enzyme, jedoch nicht ohne schädigenden Einfluß für die Endothelzelle.

Diese durch schwere Infektion induzierten Enzymsysteme können bei Nagetieren schon nach einigen Stunden nachgewiesen werden; beim Menschen ist das zeitliche Auftreten bisher nicht ausreichend dokumentiert worden. In noch nicht publizierten Studien haben wir feststellen können, daß die iNOS ab der sechsten Stunde in den epiploischen Gefäßen von Patienten mit akuter Peritonitis und Schocksymptomatik nachgewiesen werden konnte. Die vorklinische Anwendung von NOS-Inhibitoren hat beim Tier wie beim Menschen beweisen können, daß diese Enzymsysteme während der unterschiedlichen Phasen einer schweren Sepsis teilweise zum Vasomotorenkollaps beitragen [18–22]. Natürlich sind noch unzählige andere Mediatoren an diesem Vasomotorenkollaps beteiligt, von denen einige noch nicht mit Sicherheit bei Intensivpatienten identifiziert werden konnten. Unbestritten ist heute hingegen, daß die offensichtlich verminderte Ansprechbarkeit auf Katecholamine durch die Hemmung der NO-Produktion und/oder der NO-Wirkung aufgehoben werden kann. Folglich sind nun Studien über die klinische Toleranz von NOS-Hemmern und über deren tatsächliche Auswirkungen auf die Überlebensrate notwendig.

Therapeutische Richtlinien

Im Verlauf einer Infektion ist das Hauptziel der Behandlung zu verhindern, daß aus einer lokalen eine disseminierte Infektion ensteht, die von einer unangemessenen Abwehrreaktion begleitet ist. Man muß demnach mehrere Ziele gleichzeitig verfolgen:

- In erster Linie Bekämpfung aller Faktoren, die den schädigenden Einfluß auf den Organismus unterhalten,
- Verminderung aller Faktoren, die die Minderperfusion des Gewebes unterhalten oder verschlimmern (durch symptomatische Behandlung),
- Begrenzung einer unangemessenen Produktion von Entzündungsmediatoren.

Zunächst muß also die lokale Infektion bekämpft und zuletzt die Anwendung von Anti-Zytokinen diskutiert werden.

In bezug auf letztere sind schon viele klinische Studien über die Anwendung von Anti-TNF, Anti-Endotoxinen und Anti-Rezeptoren verschiedener Zytokine durchgeführt worden. Erfolgte deren Anwendung nach Einsetzen der Kreislaufstörungen, konnte keine Wirksamkeit auf die Mortalitätsrate von Patienten mit schwerer Sepsis nachgewiesen werden.

Wenn man bedenkt, daß eine schwere und/oder andauernde Verminderung des systemischen peripheren Gefäßwiderstandes mit einer erhöhten Mortalitätsrate einhergeht, dann stellt der hämodynamische Zustand des Patienten einen der wichtigsten prognostischen Faktoren dar: Somit ergibt sich als eines der Hauptbehandlungsziele die Aufrechterhaltung eines ausreichenden Perfusionsdrucks der höheren Organe und das Sicherstellen der Mindestsauerstoffversorgung der Peripherie. Unter Berücksichtigung der oben aufgeführten pathophysiologischen Zusammenhänge ist es also wichtig, eine akzeptable arterielle Sauerstoffsättigung aufrechtzuerhalten, einen ausreichenden Sauerstofftransport sicherzustellen und die regionale Durchblutung zu normalisieren. Auf die Herz-Kreislauf-Situation bezogen, sollte man demnach ein Herzzeitvolumen anstreben, das ausreicht, um einen arteriellen Blutdruck aufzubauen, der eine normale Organdurchblutung sicherstellt. Eine isolierte kardiotrope Therapie ist beim Menschen schwer durchführbar, es sei denn, das oben genannte Ziel kann allein durch den Ausgleich eines vorbestehenden Volumenmangels erreicht werden. Während der ersten 24 bis 48 Stunden nach Auftreten einer Sepsis sieht man sich jedoch häufig gezwungen, auf Pharmaka zurückzugreifen, die direkt auf die Gefäßwand wirken.

Behandlungsmöglichkeiten der akuten Kreiflaufinsuffizienz

Sobald eine normale arterielle Sauerstoffsättigung sichergestellt ist (wenn nötig, auch frühzeitig mit Hilfe mechanischer Beatmung), ist als eine der ersten Maßnahmen eine angemessene Volumensubstitution zu beginnen, um den durch das „leak syndrome" hervorgerufenen Volumenmangel auszugleichen und das Herzzeitvolumen zu normalisieren. Die Wahl des Volumenersatzmittels erfolgt zwischen kristallinen Salzlösungen und kolloidalen Plasmaersatzmitteln und orientiert sich an der Schwere des Blutdruckabfalls. Hierbei muß besonders auf das Auftreten oder die Verschlimmerung eines akuten Lungenödems durch übermäßige Volumensubstitution geachtet werden. Diese kann durch invasive Kontrolle der hämodynamischen Verlaufsparameter sicherer überwacht werden.

Substanzen, die im Augenblick zur therapeutischen Anwendung zur Verfügung stehen

Alle gefäßaktiven Substanzen, die zur Zeit für den klinischen Gebrauch zur Verfügung stehen, sind natürliche oder synthetische Katecholamine. Ihre kurzen Halbwertszeiten erfordern eine kontinuierliche intravenöse Anwendung und eine ständige Anpassung an den Volumenzustand, an die Volämie des Patienten und an seinen peripheren systemischen Gefäßwiderstand (oder an seinen arteriellen Blutdruck). Die fünf am häufigsten angewandten Substanzen sind:

- ***Dopamin:*** Es erhöht den Blutdruck durch seine gleichzeitige Wirkung auf das Herzzeitvolumen und den arteriellen Gefäßwiderstand. Niedrig dosiert besitzt es vorwiegend betamimetische Wirkung, während bei Dosierungen über 10 µg/kg/min der vasokonstriktorische Effekt überwiegt.
- ***Noradrenalin:*** Seine pharmakologische Wirkung ist hauptsächlich vom Typ Alpha; es trägt zur Steigerung sowohl des peripheren als auch des Lungengefäßwiderstands bei. Bei Dosierungen zwischen 0,05 und 0,5 µg/kg/min steigt die Herzfrequenz kaum an oder vermindert sich sogar, während das Herzzeitvolumen gleichbleibt.

- ***Adrenalin:*** Bei Dosierungen zwischen 0,05 und 0,5 µg/kg/mn wird der arterielle Blutdruck durch eine Steigerung des Herzzeitvolumens erhöht, während bei 0,5 bis 1 µg/kg/min eine direkte vasokonstriktorische Wirkung hinzukommt.
- ***Phenylephrin:*** Zwischen 0,5 bis 10 µg/kg/min wird der arterielle Blutdruck fast ausschließlich durch einen gesteigerten peripheren Gefäßwiderstand erhöht. Das Herzzeitvolumen und die Herzfrequenz können gleichzeitig ansteigen.
- ***Dobutamin:*** Bei Dosierungen zwischen 5 und 10 µg/kg/min steigt die Herzfrequenz kaum an; es erhöht den Blutdruck durch betamimetische Wirkung.

Aktive Substanzen, die zwar beim Menschen erprobt, jedoch noch nicht verfügbar sind (keine endgültige Zulassung mit eindeutiger Indikationsstellung)

- ***NO-Synthase-Hemmer*** [23]: Verschiedene Substanzgruppen sind bisher synthetisiert worden, die alle durch ihre spezifische Wirkung auf die NO-Synthase charakterisiert sind. Ihr Aktionsmodus beruht auf einer kompetitiven Hemmung des L-Arginin am Rezeptor der NO-Synthase. Einige von diesen reagieren spezifischer auf induzierbare als auf nicht induzierbare NOS (S-Methyl-Thio-Harnstoff [24]). Die ersten beim Menschen erprobten und somit die bekanntesten sind L-NMMA, L-NAME und LNNA [20–22]. Ihre Hauptaufgabe besteht darin, in die Endothelzellen und die glatten Muskelzellen einzudringen und dort die NO-Synthese zu hemmen. Somit begrenzen sie die pharmakologische NO-Wirkung auf ihre Zielmoleküle, besonders auf die Guanylat-Zyklase der Gefäßzellen. Folglich wird sowohl die in physiologischer Weise durch die elementaren NOS hervorgerufene Gefäßrelaxation als auch die im Rahmen einer schweren Sepsis durch die induzierbaren NOS ausgelöste periphere Vasodilatation aufgehoben, und die vasokonstriktorischen adrenergen Substanzen können wieder wirksam werden [19]. Ein weiterer Vorteil der NOS-Hemmer ist die Begrenzung von anfallenden NO-Metaboliten, vor allem der Peroxynitrite, welche toxisch auf die Gefäßwandzelle wirken. Ihr größter Nachteil besteht darin, daß sie die physiologische zytoprotektive NO-Basalproduktion unterdrücken, und daß sie manchmal eine starke Vasokonstriktion auslösen aufgrund des plötzlichen Überwiegens der von der Endothelzelle gleichzeitig produzierten vasodilatatorischen Substanzen.
- ***Guanylat-Zyklase-Hemmer***: Hierbei handelt es sich vor allem um Methylen-Blau, welches nicht nur eines der intrazellulären Zielmoleküle des NO hemmt [25], sondern auch unmittelbar die NO-Synthase [26]. Seine Effektivität auf

den verminderten peripheren Widerstand im septischen hyperkinetischen Schock ist eher gering, aber im Tierversuch wie in der klinischen Anwendung bewiesen [25, 27]. Sein Nutzen für die Patienten auf der Intensivstation ist bisher noch nie Gegenstand einer fundierten klinischen Studie gewesen, und somit waren wir unter den ersten, die ein ungünstiges Risiko-Nutzen-Verhältnis herausgestellt haben [25]. Es handelt sich folglich um ein Medikament mit begrenzter Einsatzmöglichkeit und seine Anwendung ist zur Zeit kaum zu empfehlen.

Therapeutische Perspektiven

In nicht allzu naher Zukunft wird man die schwere Infektion als Angriff auf den Zellkern betrachten. Einige vorläufige experimentelle Ergebnisse lassen uns in der Tat an eine mögliche Einsetzbarkeit neuer therapeutischer Substanzen denken, wie zum Beispiel gegensinnige Oligonukleotide, die gegen die mRNA der induzierbaren NOS gerichtet sind [28]: Beim mit LPS vorbehandelten Tier haben diese Substanzen die Fähigkeit bewiesen, dem Verlust der arteriellen Noradrenalin-Sensibilität vorzubeugen. Diese Art pharmakologischer Substanzen stellt demnach eine Hoffnung dar, die durch klinische Studien bestätigt werden muß. Übrigens sind auch andere Forschungszweige Grundlage neuer Studien, wie die Hemmer des NF-κB oder der Poly-(ADP)-Ribosyl-Polymerase [29, 30], die eine bedeutende Verminderung der akuten Kreislaufinsuffizienz bei Nagetieren gezeigt haben.

Therapeutische Indikationen

Mehrere Konsensus-Konferenzen sind zu ähnlichen Schlufolgerungen in bezug auf die therapeutischen Indikationsstellungen im Verlauf einer Infektion mit Gefäßreaktion gekommen [31, 32].

Übereinstimmungen

Da in jedem Falle eine Hypovolämie bei diesen Patienten vorliegt, besteht ein breiter Konsens im Hinblick auf die Anwendung von Volumenersatzmitteln an erster Stelle. Über die Art des zu verwendenden Therapeutikums ist man sich zwar noch nicht einig, es scheint jedoch vernünftiger, so wenig wie möglich auf Substanzen menschlicher Herkunft (Albumine) zurückzugreifen, als vielmehr synthetische Lösungen wie Kolloide oder HES vorzuziehen. Den Inhalt vieler Diskussionen stellt auch das Ausmaß der Volumensubstitution dar, welches um so schwieriger wird, wenn keine invasiven hämodynamischen Kontrollen durchgeführt werden. Oberste Priorität bleibt in jedem Fall das Sicherstellen eines ausreichenden arteriellen Blutdrucks und das Herstellen einer effektiven Diurese, welche Ausdruck einer adäquaten peripheren Durchblutung ist. Vorgesehen ist, die Volumensubstitution beim Erwachsenen mit 500 ml einer kolloidalen Lösung blind zu beginnen. Bei unverändert niedrigem Blutdruck kann diese unter Kontrolle des zentralen Venendruckes oder wenn möglich unter Echokardiographiekontrolle wiederholt werden.

Die kontinuierliche Dopamininfusion stellt die zweite Therapiemodalität dar: Diese hat nicht immer eine für die Nierendurchblutung ausreichende Blutdruckerhöhung zu Folge; in diesem Falle ist man gezwungen, auf Noradrenalin zurückzugreifen, dessen Anwendung eine hämodynamische Überwachung mittels eines pulmonal-arteriellen Swan-Ganz-Katheters erfordert. Somit wird es also möglich, zunächst eine ausgewogene Normovolämie herzustellen, um dann jene klinischen Situationen abzugrenzen, in denen das periphere Kreislaufversagen die zentrale Herzinsuffizienz überwiegt. Im diesem Falle ist es ratsam, die Behandlung mit einer Kombination von Noradrenalin und Dobutamin fortzusetzten, während bei Überwiegen der Herzinsuffizienz die Anwendung von Adrenalin indiziert ist.

Unstimmigkeiten

In Wirklichkeit erscheint mangelnde Übereinstimmung in der Behandlung des Kreislaufversagens bei schwerer Sepsis erst dann, wenn alle oben gennanten Behandlungsmethoden nicht zu einer Verbesserung der Kreislauf- und Stoffwechsellage (Normalisierung der Laktazidose) führen. Es handelt sich also um die Frage, ob innovative Pharmaka wie die NOS-Hemmer zur Aufrechterhaltung des Blutdrucks und zur Verminderung der Mortalität eingesetzt werden sollten. Nach aktuellem Wissensstand können wir diese ohne konsequent durchgeführte wissenschaftliche Studien nicht empfehlen. Man muß zwar zugestehen, daß diese Substanzen ihre pharmakologische Wirksamkeit bewiesen haben, sie jedoch den späteren Tod durch Multiorganversagen nicht signifikant vermindern konnten.

Ergebnisse

Trotz der zur Verfügung stehenden Therapiemöglichkeiten, um den Vasomotorenkollaps, der im Rahmen einer schwerer Infektion an der Gefäßwand selbst ausgelöst wird, entgegenzuwirken, bleibt die unkontrollierte Schocksituation die Haupttodesursache in der Initialphase einer schweren Sepsis. Die Ursache der Mortalität scheint in den letzten Jahren eher das Multiorganversagen zu sein, welches wahrscheinlich durch die Fortschritte in der symptomatischen Intensivmedizin erklärt werden kann. Auf unserer intensiv-medizinischen Abteilung ist die Gesamtsterblichkeit mit 50% konstant geblieben; man muß jedoch darauf hinweisen, daß sich unter den Patienten ein wachsender Anteil schwer immunsupprimierter Patienten befindet.

Schlußfolgerung

Der in der Intensivmedizin angetroffenen schweren Infektion liegt ein dynamischer Prozeß zugrunde, in dem jede Phase die ihr angemessene Behandlung erfordert. Lebenswichtig ist die symptomatische Behandlung der auftretenden Gefäßreaktionen mit dem Ziel, einen ausreichenden Perfusionsdruck für eine effektive Organdurchblutung aufrechtzuerhalten. Falls diese durch Volumensubstitution allein nicht sichergestellt werden kann, ist es unumgänglich, auf vasoaktive Substanzen zurückzugreifen, deren Art und Dosierung an die hämodynamischen Parameter anzupassen sind. In Übereinstimmung mit den Empfehlungen vielfältiger Experten-Kommissionen setzen wir eine Kombinationsbehandlung ein, bestehend aus einem positiv inotropen Anteil in Verbindung mit einem Vasokonstriktor (Adrenalin oder Noradrenalin). Falls sich die Aufhebung des Vasomotorenkollaps trotz Normalisierung der biologischen Parameter als unmöglich erweist, bleiben uns nur innovative Therapiealternativen (NO-Synthase-Hemmer). In naher Zukunft müssen Therapiealternativen berücksichtigt werden, die in der Lage sind, die Gensynthese und die Genexpression im Rahmen einer komplexen Abwehrreaktion zu modulieren, ungeachtet der Art des zugrunde liegenden schädigenden Agens.

Literatur

1. Suffredini AF, Fromm RE, Parker MM, Brenner M, Kovacs JA, Wesley RA, Parrillo JE (1989) The cardiovascular response of normal humans to the administration of endotoxin. N Engl J Med 3:280–286
2. Parrillo JE, Parker MM, Natanson C, Suffredini AF, Danner RL, Cunnion RE, Ognibene FP (1990) Septic shock in humans. Ann Intern Med 113:227–242
3. Thijs LG, Groeneveld ABJ (1988) Peripheral circulation in septic shock. ACP 2:203–214
4. Thiemermann C, Vane J (1990) Inhibition of nitric oxide synthesis reduces the hypotension induced by bacterial lipopolysaccharide in the rat in vivo. Eur J Pharmacol 182:591–595
5. Paya D, Stoclet JC (1995) Involvement of bradykinin and nitric oxide in the early hemodynamic effects of lipopolysaccharide in rats. Shock 3:376–379
6. Ghosh S, Liu MS (1983) Changes in -adrenergic receptors in dog livers during endotoxic shock. J Surg Res 34:239–245
7. Ball HA, Cook JA, Wise WC, Halushka PV (1986) Role of thromboxane, prostaglandins and leukotrienes in endotoxic and septic shock. Intensive Care Med 12:116–126
8. Fink MP, MacVittie TJ, Casey LC (1984) Inhibition of prostaglandin synthesis restores normal hemodynamics in canine hyperdynamic sepsis. Ann Surg 200:619–626
9. Sigurdsson GH, Youssel HAF, Banic A (1993) Effects of ketoprofen on respiratory and circulatory changes in endotoxic shock. Intensive Care Med 19:333-339
10. Glauser MP (1996) The inflammatory cytokines. New developments in the pathophysiology and treatment of septic shock. Drugs 52:9–17
11. Curzen NP, Griffiths MJD, Evas TW (1994) Role of the endothelium in modulating the vascular response to sepsis. Clin Sci 86:359–374
12. Billiau A, Vanderkerckhove F (1991) Cytokines and their interactions with other inflammatory mediators in the pathogenesis of sepsis and septic shock. Eur J Clin Invest 21:559–573
13. Tobias PS, Mathison JC, Ulevitch RJ (1988) A family of lipopolysaccharide binding proteins involved in responses to gram-negative sepsis. J Biol Chem 263:13479–13481
14. Blackwell TS, Christman JW (1997) The role of nuclear factor-kappa B in cytokine gene regulation. Am J Respir Cell Molecular Biol 17:3–9
15. Stoclet JC, Fleming I, Gray G, Julou-Schaeffer G, Schneider F, Schott C, Schott Ch, Parratt JR (1993) Nitric oxide and endotoxemia. Circulation 87:V77–V80
16. Yet SF, Pellacani A, Patterson C, Tan L, Folta SC, Foster L, Lee WS, Hsieh CM, Perella MA (1997) Induction of heme oxygenase-1 expression in vascular smooth muscle cells: a link to endotoxin shock. J Biol Chem 272:4295–4301
17. Song SK, Karl IE, Ackerman JJH, Hotchkiss RS (1993) Incrased intracellular Ca2+: a critical link in the pathophysiology of sepsis? Proc Natl Acad Sci USA 90:3933–3937
18. Julou-Schaeffer G, Gray GA, Fleming I, Schott C, Parratt JR, Stoclet JC (1990) Loss of vascular responsiveness induced by endotoxin involves L-arginine pathway. Am J Physiol (Heart Circ Phy) 259:H1038–H1043
19. Schneider F, Bucher F, Schott C, André A, Julou-Schaeffer G, Stoclet JC (1994) Effect of bacterial lipopolysaccharide on function of rat small femoral arteries. Am J Physiol (Heart Circ Phy) 266:H191–H198
20. Petros A, Bennett D, Vallance P (1991) Effect of nitric synthase inhibitors on hypotension in patients with septic shock. Lancet 338:1557–1558

21. Petros A, Lamb G, Leone A, Moncada S, Bennett D, Vallance P (1994) Effects of a nitric oxide synthase inhibitor in humans with septic shock. Cardiovasc Res 28:34–39
22. Gomez-Jimenez J, Salgado A, Mourelle M et al. (1995) L-arginine – nitric oxide pathway in endotoxemia and human septic shock. Crit Care Med 23:253–258
23. Rees DD, Palmer RMJ, Schulz R, Hodson HF, Moncada S (1990) Characterization of three inhibitors of endothelial nitric oxide synthase in vitro and in vivo. Br J Pharmacol 101:746–752
24. Rees DD, Palmer RMJ, Schulz R, Hodson HF, Moncada S (1993) Aminoguanidine selectively inhibits inducible nitric oxide synthase. Br J Pharmacol 110:963–968
25. Schneider F, Lutun Ph, Hasselmann M, Stoclet JC, Tempé JD (1992) Methylene blue increases systemic vascular resistance in human septic shock. Intensive Care Med 18: 309–311
26. MacEvoy G, Litvak K, Welsh O (1994) Methylene blue. American Hospital Formulary Services drug information 1994. American Society of Hospital Pharmacists, pp 2118–2119
27. Paya D, Gray GA, Stoclet JC (1993) Effects of methylene blue on blood pressure and reactivity to norepinephrine in endotoxemic rats. J Cardiovasc Pharmacol 21:926–930
28. Hoque AM, Papapetropoulos A, Venema RC, Catravas JD, Fuchs LC (1998) Effects of antisense oligonucleotide to iNOS on hemodynamic and vascular changes induced by LPS. Amer J Physiol (Heart Circ Phy) 44:H1078–H1083
29. Taylor BS, Devera ME, Ganster RW, Wang Q, Shapiro RA, Morris SM, Billiar TR, Geller DA (1998) Multiple NF-Kappa B enhancer elements regulate cytokine induction of the human inducible nitric oxide synthase gene. J Biol Chem 273:15148–15156
30. Wray GM, Hinds CJ, Thiemermann C (1998) Effects of inhibitors of poly (ADP-ribose) -synthetase activity on hypotension and multiple organ dysfunction caused by endotoxin. Shock 10:13–19
31. XVe Conférence de Consensus en Réanimation et Médecine d'Urgence (1996) Utilisation des catécholamines au cours du choc septique. Réa Urg 5:441–450
32. Consensus Conference (1998) Resuscitation of patients in septic shock. Int Care World 15:72–83

Niereninsuffizienz bei Sepsis

K.-U. Eckardt

Akute Niereninsuffizienz bis hin zum oligo-anurischen Nierenversagen ist eine der für eine Sepsis typischen Organfunktionsstörungen, die neben der systemischen Entzündungsreaktion das klinische Bild und die Prognose septischer Patienten bestimmen [28]. Umgekehrt spielt systemische Inflammation eine wesentliche Rolle in der bei Intensivpatienten meistens multifaktoriellen Pathogenese des akuten Nierenversagens (ANV). In dieser kurzen Übersicht werden einige Evidenzen für die klinische Bedeutung eines ANV bei Sepsis zusammengefaßt und die Pathomechanismen skizziert, durch die es bei Sepsis zu einer Einschränkung der Nierenfunktion kommt.

Inzidenz und prognostische Bedeutung

Der Definition von SIRS, Sepsis, schwerer Sepsis und septischem Schock [1] liegt das Konzept zugrunde, daß es sich dabei nicht um unterschiedliche Krankheitsbilder, sondern um verschiedene Stadien einer systemischen Entzündungsreaktion handelt. Diese Hypothese konnte durch eine große prospektive Untersuchung bestätigt werden, in der die klinische Progression von SIRS bis hin zum septischem Schock belegt wurde [31]. Die dabei erhobenen Daten zu Organfunktionsstörungen zeigen, daß die Inzidenz eines ANV im Rahmen dieser Progression von unter 10 auf knapp 50% zunimmt (Tabelle 1). Ob das ANV eine Bedeutung für die mit der Progredienz des inflammatorischen Bildes verbundene Zunahme der Mortalität hat, ist nicht geklärt. Da ein Nierenversagen aber in anderen untersuchten Kollektiven als ein unabhängiger Risikofaktor identifiziert wurde [9, 19], ist ein über die anderen Auswirkungen der Sepsis hinausgehender prognostisch ungünstiger Einfluß der Nierenfunktionsstörung nicht auszuschließen. Sicher ist, daß die Prognose von Patienten mit ANV bei Sepsis deutlich schlechter ist als die von Patienten mit Nierenversagen aus anderen Ur-

Tabelle 1. Inzidenz von akutem Nierenversagen (ANV) im Vergleich zu ARDS und disseminierter Gerinnung (DIC) mit progredientem Schweregrad systemischer Inflammation

	ARDS (%)	DIC (%)	ANV (%)	Mortalität (%)
SIRS				
zwei Kriterien	2	8	9	7
drei Kriterien	3	15	13	10
vier Kriterien	6	19	19	17
Sepsis				16
Kultur-positiv	6	16	19	
Kultur-negativ	3	20	5	
Schwere Sepsis				20
Kultur-positiv	8	18	23	
Kultur-negativ	4	17	16	
Septischer Schock				46
Kultur-positiv	18	38	51	
Kultur-negativ	18	38	38	

Ergebnisse einer prospektiven Untersuchung an mehr als 3700 Patienten [31]

sachen. In einer kürzlich in Frankreich durchgeführten Multizenterstudie mit 360 Intensivpatienten mit ANV war Sepsis einer von sieben unabhängigen Mortalitätsprädiktoren [5]. Die Krankenhausmortalität von septischen Patienten betrug in diesem Kollektiv 75% im Vergleich zu 45% bei Patienten mit ANV ohne Sepsis [24]. Interessanterweise zeigte eine Vergleichsuntersuchung über Begleiterkrankungen und Mortalität von Patienten mit ANV im Zeitraum von 1977–79 und 1991–92 an der Mayo-Klinik, daß sich die ungünstige Prognose von septischen Patienten mit ANV in dem untersuchten Zeitraum auch nicht verändert hat, obwohl die Krankenhausmortalität von Patienten mit ANV insgesamt deutlich gesunken ist [23].

Pathomechanismen

Aus den o.g. epidemiologischen Beobachtungen ergibt sich vor allem die Frage, wodurch es mit Progredienz einer systemischen Inflammation zu einer zunehmend häufigeren und schwereren Beeinträchtigung der Nierenfunktion kommt. Die Konzepte dazu sind nach wie vor lückenhaft und stützen sich vor allem auf die Ergebnisse von Tierexperimenten. Obwohl deren Übertragbarkeit

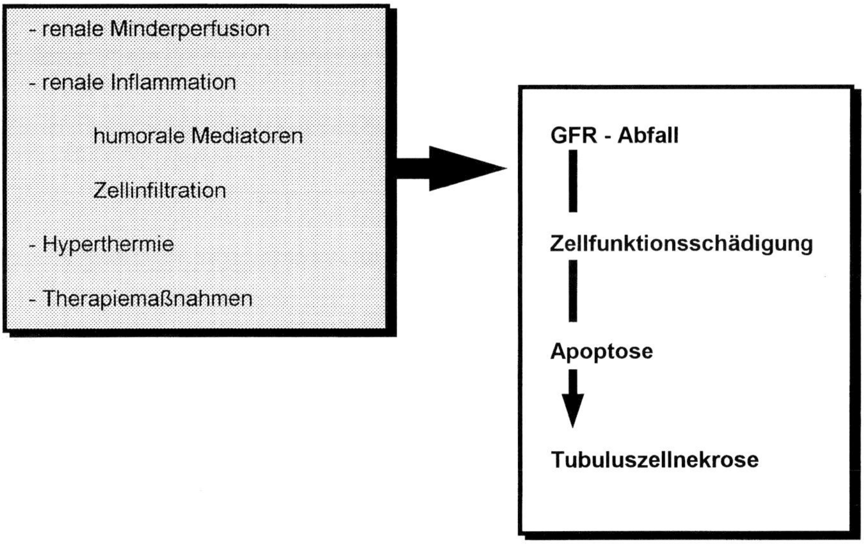

Abb. 1. Pathomechanismen einer Nierenfunktionsstörung bei Sepsis

auf die klinische Situation beim Menschen immer hinterfragt werden muß, konnten dadurch zahlreiche Teilaspekte identifiziert werden, die vermutlich in unterschiedlicher Ausprägung und Abfolge einen Einfluß auf die Nierenfunktion septischer Patienten haben (Abb. 1). Manche dieser Pathomechanismen sind vermutlich auch nicht speziell oder ausschließlich für die Niere relevant, sondern gleichermaßen an der Entstehung anderer Organfunktionsstörungen beteiligt.

Renale Minderperfusion

Eine Störung der renalen Durchblutung kommt im Rahmen aller Formen eines ANV vermutlich eine wesentliche pathophysiologische Bedeutung zu. Allerdings ist die Nierenperfusion, soweit dazu Daten vorliegen, auch bei anurischen Patienten nur um etwa die Hälfte reduziert, so daß zusätzliche Mechanismen vorliegen müssen, die zum Abfall der glomerulären Filtrationsrate (GFR) bis hin zum kompletten Verlust der Urinproduktion führen [12, 20].

Auch bei der Sepsis kommt es vermutlich in den meisten Fällen zu einer renalen Minderperfusion [36]. Damit unterscheidet sich die renale Hämodynamik von der der meisten anderen Gefäßgebiete, in denen es zu einer Abnahme des Gefäßwiderstandes und einer Zunahme der Gesamtperfusion kommt. Beim Menschen liegen nur wenige Daten über Veränderungen des renalen Blutflusses im Verlauf eines ANV vor, da die für die Blutflußmessung üblicherweise verwandten Clearancetechniken bei (Oligo-) Anurie naturgemäß nicht durchführbar sind. Mit Hilfe von Thermodilutionskathetern, die in die Nierenvene eingeführt wurden, konnte aber zumindest bei einer kleinen Gruppe von Patienten der renale Blutfluß während und nach einer hyperdynamen septischen Kreislaufsituation gemessen werden [4]. Im Gegenstatz zum systemischen Gesamtwiderstand, war der renale Widerstand dabei nicht erniedrigt und der renale Blutfluß signifikant reduziert.

In tierexperimentellen Untersuchungen konnte durch simultane Perfusionsmessungen verschiedener Organe mit Mikrosphärentechniken bestätigt werden, daß die Niere damit eine Sonderstellung einnimmt. Im Gegensatz zur Reduktion der renalen Perfusion nimmt die Durchblutung anderer Organe wie Herz, Gehirn und Magen zu oder bleibt zumindest, wie in Leber, Muskulatur und Haut, weitgehend konstant [8]. Lediglich in der Milz wurde unter Infusion von E. coli bei Affen ebenfalls eine Abnahme der Durchblutung nachgewiesen [8]. Andere Untersuchungen bei Affen haben darüber hinaus gezeigt, daß es unter Infusion mit E. coli zu charakteristischen zeitabhängigen Veränderungen der renalen Perfusion kommt und der Abfall von renalem Plasmafluß und GFR sich 2 Stunden nach einer E.-coli-Infusion vorübergehend bessert [32], ohne daß die Ursachen dieser Perfusionsschwankungen klar sind. Bei Hunden wurde gezeigt, daß die Veränderungen der renalen Hämodynamik unter Endotoxininfusion mit einem Abfall des Sauerstoffpartialdruckes im Nierenkortex und einer Abnahme des renalen Sauerstoffverbrauches einhergehen [14].

Potentielle Mediatoren renaler Vasokonstriktion

Aus der im Vergleich zu anderen Gefäßgebieten divergenten renalen Hämodynamik ergibt sich die Frage, wodurch eine renale Vasokonstriktion bei septischen Krankheitsbildern vermittelt wird. Tierexperimentelle Untersuchungen haben zeigen können, daß es bereits unter Endotoxindosen, die noch zu keiner Beeinträchtigung des systemischen Blutdruckes führen, zu einer Verminderung von renalem Blutfluß und GFR kommt [11,36]. Interessanterweise führen Endotoxinkonzentrationen, die dabei im Plasma erreicht werden, in isoliert perfundierten Nieren aber zu keiner Beeinträchtigung der Hämodynamik und Funktion [11]. Diese wichtigen Befunde weisen darauf hin, daß Endotoxin nicht direkt, sondern über außerhalb der Niere gebildete Mediatoren die Nierenfunktion beeinflußt. Die Liste von Substanzen, die bei der Vermittlung einer renalen Vasokonstriktion möglicherweise eine Rolle spielen, ist lang und umfaßt u.a. Katecholamine, Produkte des Arachidonsäuremetabolismus, Komponenten des Renin-Angiotensin-Systems, Zytokine, Endothelin und Stickstoffmonoxid (Tabelle 2). Obwohl es unter zahlreichen experimentellen Bedingungen möglich ist, durch Applikation einzelner Substanzen und ihrer Agonisten und Antagonisten Hinweise für ihre jeweilige Bedeutung zu erarbeiten, ist es unter klinischen Bedingungen vermutlich nicht die Überproduktion oder das Fehlen einzelner Mediatoren, sondern eine Dysbalance vasokonstriktorischer und vasodilatatorischer Substanzen insgesamt, die zur renalen Perfusionsminderung führt. Die präferentiell renale Vasokonstriktion bei gleichzeitiger Dilatation anderer Gefäßgebiete läßt sich theoretisch dadurch erklären, daß das Verhältnis vasokonstriktorischer und vasodilatatorischer Effektoren in der Niere anders ist als in anderen Organen und/oder die renalen Widerstandsgefäße aufgrund entsprechender Rezeptoren und Signaltransduktionsmechanismen eher im Sinne einer Vasokonstriktion reagieren. Auf Endothelin beispielsweise, ein vasokonstriktorisches Peptid aus 21 Aminosäuren, dessen pathophysiologische Bedeutung in vielen Zusammenhängen diskutiert wird, reagieren die renalen Gefäße deutlich sensibler als die Gefäße anderer Organe [17]. Erhöhte Plasma-Endothelinspiegel bei Patienten mit Sepsis, die invers mit der Kreatininclearance korreliert sind [35], und die positiven Effekte von Endothelinantikörpern auf die GFR von Tieren unter Endotoxininfusion [2] weisen auf eine Bedeutung von Endothelin für das Sepsis-assoziierte Nierenversagen hin.

Konstitutiv produziertes Stickstoffmonoxid (NO) trägt als Vasodilatator zur physiologischen Regulation des Gefäßtonus bei. Es ist denkbar, aber bislang nicht bewiesen, daß eine lokale Verminderung dieser konstitutiven NO-Produktion zum Anstieg des renalen Widerstandes bei Sepsis beiträgt. Umgekehrt trägt

Tabelle 2. Potentielle Mediatoren renaler Vasokonstriktion bei Sepsis

• Arginin-Vasopressin	[33]
• Angiotensin II	[33]
• Adenosin	[10]
• Endothelin	[2, 16, 35]
• Thromboxan A2	[3, 6]
• Leukotriene	[3, 6]
• Zytokine	[16, 18]
• NO	[15, 27]

eine vermehrte NO-Produktion durch die durch Lipopolysaccharid oder Zytokine induzierbare NO-Synthase vermutlich wesentlich zur Vasodilatation und arteriellen Hypotension beim septischen Schock bei. Durch polymerisiertes Hämoglobin, einen potentiellen Scavanger von NO, ließen sich in einem Endotoxinschock-Modell der Ratte Kreislauf- und Nierenfunktion normalisieren [15].

Neben funktionellen Veränderungen des renalen Gefäßtonus können bei schwerer Sepsis auch Mikrothromben zur Minderperfusion beitragen [34].

Renale Inflammation

Daß zahlreiche Entzündungsmediatoren potentielle Mediatoren renaler Vasokonstriktion sind, weist bereits auf die enge Verknüpfung zwischen der hämodynamischen und der inflammatorischen Reaktion der Niere hin. Daneben spielt die Infiltration von Granulozyten und Monozyten eine wichtige Rolle für die renale Funktionsstörung. Die in die Niere eingewanderten Entzündungszellen tragen wesentlich zur lokalen Produktion von inflammatorischen und im weitesten Sinne zytotoxischen Substanzen bei. Zwar können auch zytopenische Patienten ein Nierenversagen entwickeln, aber in vielen experimentellen Modellen eines ANV läßt sich die Nierenfunktion durch Hemmung der Leukozyteninfiltration günstig beeinflussen [29]. Wie in allen Organen spielt die Interaktion mit Endothelzellen eine Schlüsserolle bei der Gewebsinfiltration von Granulozyten und Monozyten. Adhäsionsmoleküle auf Endothelzellen binden Integrine weißer Blutkörperchen und ermöglichen so den Kontakt dieser Zellen mit der Gefäßwand und die anschließende Durchwanderung. Die Expression der Adhäsionsmoleküle ICAM-1 und VCAM-1, die nach der Strömungsverlangsamung für das Anhaften von Granulozyten und Monozyten an Endothelzellen verantwortlich sind, wird durch Zytokine, wie z. B. TNF α, und auch durch Anstiege des periendothelialen Sauerstoffpartialdruckes stimuliert [7, 37]. Perfusionsschwankungen in der Niere im Rahmen septischer Zustände können zu solchen Anstiegen der lokalen Oxygenierung führen.

Besondere Bedeutung hat im Rahmen systemischer Entzündungsreaktionen, daß nicht nur Effekte auf Endothelzellen, sondern auch eine Aktivierung zirkulierender Granulozyten deren Infiltration in das Gewebe begünstigt. Dieser Mechanismus konnte in isoliert perfundierten Nieren belegt werden, in denen eine vorangegangene renale Ischämie und Vorstimulation von Granulozyten im Perfusat potenzierende Effekte auf die Neutrophilenretention und parallel dazu auf den Abfall der renalen Filtrationsrate hatten [22].

Hyperthermie

Neben direkten renalen Effekten von solublen und zellulären Mediatoren kann eine systemische Entzündungsreaktion die Nierenfunktion möglicherweise auch indirekt beinträchtigen. Beispielsweise gibt es experimentelle Evidenzen dafür, daß das Ausmaß einer Nierenschädigung durch temporären Nierenarterienverschluß temperaturabhängig ist [38]. Der Anstieg von Kreatinin und Harnstoff im Plasma war bei diesen Untersuchungen bei Ratten nach Nierenischämie unter Hypothermie geringer und unter mäßiger Hyperthermie (38–39 °C) signifikant größer als unter Normothermie.

Nierenschädigung durch Therapiemaßnahmen

Neben den verschiedenen Auswirkungen der systemischen Inflammation bis hin zur Sepsis können auch die notwendigen Therapiemaßnahmen einen ungünstigen Einfluß auf die Nierenfunktion haben. Die renalen Gefäße reagieren beispielsweise sensibel auf Norepinephrin, so daß sich die renale Perfusion verschlechtern kann, wenn der arterielle Mitteldruck durch Gabe dieses Katecholamins angehoben wird. Wie weit die renale Perfusion durch Dopamin und verwandte Substanzen gesteigert werden kann, ist nach wie vor umstritten [26]. Ähnlich wie in anderen Situationen ist auch bei septischen Patienten die positive Wirkung von Dopamin auf die Nierenfunktion nicht ausreichend belegt [13].

Neben Katecholaminen tragen Aminoglykosidantibiotika häufig zum Nierenversagen septischer Patienten bei. Die Mechanismen der Nephrotoxizität dieser Substanzen sind nach wie vor nicht völlig geklärt. Interessante experimentelle Hinweise gibt es für einen synergistischen nephrotoxischen Effekt von Gentamycin und gram-negativer Bakteriämie [39].

Nichtletale Funktionsstörung, Apoptose und Nekrose von Tubuluszellen

Bei allen Formen des ANV geht man davon aus, daß es ein Kontinuum der Schädigung von unmittelbar reversiblen Funktionsstörungen bis hin zur Tubuluszellnekrose gibt. Insbesondere im angloamerikanischen Sprachgebrauch wird der Begriff „acute tubular necrosis" häufig nahezu synonym mit dem Begriff „ANV" gebraucht. Histologische Untersuchungen der Nierenstruktur bei Patienten mit ANV gibt es nur wenige, aber die vorhandenen Befunde zeigen im allgemeinen keine sehr ausgedehnten Nekrosen. Man muß deshalb davon ausgehen, daß neben Nekrosen als schwerster Form der Nierenschädigung vor allem subletale Zellfunktionsstörungen, z.B. über den Verlust der Zelladhäsion und die Abschilferung von Epithelien in das Tubuluslumen, für den Nierenfunktionsverlust eine wichtige Rolle spielen [20, 30]. Außerdem gibt es zunehmend Hinweise dafür, daß neben der Nekrose von Tubulusepithelien auch die Apoptose dieser Zellen beim ANV eine wichtige Rolle spielt. Dabei scheinen bestimmte zellschädigende Einflüsse nicht spezifisch entweder Nekrose oder Apoptose zu induzieren, sondern verschiedene zellschädigende Faktoren können in Abhängigkeit von ihrem Schweregrad zu subletaler reversibler Schädigung, Apoptose oder Nekrose führen [21].

In Zusammenhang mit Sepsis ist relevant, daß im Tiermodell in vivo und in vitro Lipopolysaccharid und Zytokine wie TNF α eine Apoptose von Tubulusepithelien durch Induktion des Fas-Rezeptors und seines Liganden induzieren können [25].

Zusammenfassung

Die Inzidenz des akuten Nierenversagens nimmt bei Patienten mit zunehmendem Schweregrad systemischer Inflammation progredient zu, und bei etwa der Hälfte aller Intensivpatienten mit akutem Nierenversagen spielt Sepsis eine Rolle in der Pathogenese der Nierenfunktionsstörung. Im Gegensatz zur hyperdynamen Kreislaufsituation mit Abfall des systemischen Gesamtwiderstandes ist die Perfusion der Niere bei Sepsis vermindert, was für die Entstehung des Nierenversagens septischer Patienten vermutlich eine wichtige Rolle spielt. Zahlreiche Mediatoren können dazu beitragen, daß in der Niere die Balance zwischen vasokonstriktorischen und vasodilatatorischen Einflüssen gestört ist. Warum die renalen Widerstandsgefäße bei systemischer Inflammation anders reagieren als die der meisten anderen Organe, ist aber nicht klar. Neben den hämodynamischen Effekten spielt vor allem die Infiltration der Niere mit aktivierten Entzündungszellen eine wesentliche Rolle für die Funktionseinschränkung. Daneben können auch Therapiemaßnahmen, wie beispielsweise Katecholamine, die die renale Vasokonstriktion verstärken, oder nephrotoxische Antibiotika die Entstehung eines Nierenversagens bei Sepsis begünstigen. Fortschritte in der Behandlung des ANV bei Sepsis wurden in den letzten Jahrzehnten vor allem durch Weiterentwicklung der Nierenersatztherapie, insbesondere in Form von kontinuierlichen Verfahren erreicht. Die pharmakologische oder auch gentechnologische Beeinflussung der Mediatorsysteme, die ein ANV bei Sepsis vermutlich induzieren und aufrechterhalten, ist bislang nur tierexperimentell erfolgreich. Sie eröffnet aber Optionen, die zukünftig möglicherweise auch klinische Relevanz erlangen können.

Literatur

1. American College of Chest Physicians – Society of Critical Care Medicine Consenus Conference (1992) Definitions for sepsis and organ failure and guidelines for the use of innovative therapies in sepsis. Crit Care Med 20:864–875
2. Badr KF (1992) Sepsis-associated renal vasoconstriction: potential targets for future therapy. Am J Kid Dis 20:207–213
3. Badr KF, Kelley VE, Rennke HG, Brenner BM (1986) Roles of thromboxane A2 and leukotrienes in endotoxin-induced acute renal failure. Kidney Int 30:474–480
4. Brenner M, Schaer GL, Mallory DL, Suffredini AF, Parillo JE (1999) Detection of renal blood flow abnormalities in septic and critically ill patients using a newly designed indwelling thermodilution renal vein catheter. Chest 98:170–179
5. Brivet FG, Kleinknecht DJ, Loirat P, Landais PJM (1996) Acute renal failure in intensive care units – causes, outcome, and prognostic factors of hospital mortality: a prospective, multicenter trial. Crit Care Med 24:192–198
6. Burnier M, Waeber B, Aubert JF, Nussberger J, Brunner HR (1988) Effects of nonhypotensive endotoxemia in conscious rats: role of prostaglandins. Am J Physiol 254: H509–H516
7. Carlos TM, Harlan JM (1996) Leukocyte-endothelial adhesion molecules. Blood 84: 2068–2101
8. Carroll GC, Snyder JV (1982) Hyperdynamic severe intravascular sepsis depends on fluid administration in cynomolgus monkey. Am J Physiol 243:R131–R141
9. Chertow GM, Levy EM, Hammermeister KE, Grover F, Daley J (1998) Independent association between acute renal failure and mortality following cardiac surgery. Am J Med 104:343–348
10. Churchill PC, Bidani AK, Schwartz MM (1987) Renal effects of endotoxin in the male rat. Am J Physiol 253:F244–F250
11. Cohen JJ, Black AJ, Wertheim SJ (1990) Direct effects of endotoxin on the function of the isolated perfused rat kidney. Kidney Int 37:1219–1226
12. Conger JD, Briner VA, Schrier RW (1992) Acute renal failure: pathogenesis, diagnosis, and management. In: Schrier RW (ed) Renal and electrolyte disorders, 4th ed. Little, Brown and Company, Boston Toronto London, pp 495–538
13. Denton MD, Chertow GM, Brady HR (1995) „Renal-dose" dopamine for the treatment of acute reanl failure: scientific rationale, experimental studies and clinical trials. Kidney Int 49:4–14
14. Gullichsen E, Nelimarkka O, Halkola L, Niinikoski J (1989) Renal oxygenation in endotoxin shock in dogs. Crit Care Med 17:547–550
15. Heneka MT, Löschmann PA, Osswald H (1997) Polymerized hemoglobin restores cardiovascular and kidney function in endotoxin-induced shock in the rat. J Clin Invest 99: 47–54

16. Kohan DE (1994) Role of endothelin and tumour necrosis factor in the renal response to sepsis. Nephrol Dial Transpl 9 (Suppl 4): 73–77
17. Kohan DE (1997) Endothelins in the normal and diseased kidney. Am J Kid Dis 29: 2–26
18. Koltai M, Pirotzky E, Braquet P (1994) PAF-cytokine autocatalytic feed-back network in septic shock: involvement in acute renal failure. Nephrol Dial Transpl 9 (Suppl 4): 69–72
19. Levy EM, Viscoli CM, Horwitz RI (1996) The effect of acute renal failure on mortality. JAMA 275: 1489–1494
20. Lieberthal W (1997) Biology of acute renal failure: therapeutic implications. Kidney Int 52: 1102–1115
21. Lieberthal W, Levine JS (1996) Mechanisms of apoptosis and its potential role in renal tubular epithelial cell injury. Am J Physiol 271: F477–F488
22. Linas SL, Whittenburg D, Parsons PE, Repine JE (1995) Ischemia increases neutrophil retention and worsens acute renal failure: role of oxygen metabolites and ICAM 1. Kidney Int 48: 1584–1591
23. McCarthy JT (1996) Prognosis of patients with acute renal failure in the intensive care unit: a tale of two eras. Mayo Clin Proc 71: 117–126
24. Neveu H, Kleinknecht D, Brivet F, Loirat P, Landais P (1996) Prognostic factors in acute renal failure due to sepsis. Results of a prospective multicentre study. Nephrol Dial Transpl 11: 293–299
25. Ortiz-Arduan A, Danoff TM, Kalluri R, Gonzalez-Cuadrado S, Karp SL, Elkon K, Egido J, Neilson E (1996) Regulation of Fas and Fas ligand expression in cultured murine renal cells and in the kidney during endotoxemia. Am J Physiol 271: F1193–F1201
26. Palsson J, Ricksten SE, Houltz E, Lundin S (1997) Effects of dopamine, dopexamine and dobutamine on renal excretory function during experimental sepsis in conscious rats. Acta Anaesthesiol Scand 41: 392–398
27. Papadimitriou M, Economidou D, Vakianis P, Raidis C, Vrettos M, Margari P, Leontsini M (1994) Effect of inhibition of nitiric oxide synthase in acute renal failure due to endotoxin shock in dogs. Nephrol Dial Transpl 9 (Suppl. 4): 82–87
28. Parrillo JE (1993) Pathogenetic mechanisms of septic shock. New Engl J Med 328: 1471–1477
29. Rabb H, O'Meara YM, Maderna P, Coleman P, Brady HR (1997) Leukocytes, cell adhesion molecules and ischemic acute renal failure. Kidney Int 51: 1463–1468
30. Racusen LC (1992) Alterations in tubular epithelial cell adhesion and mechanisms of acute renal failure. Lab Invest 67: 158–165
31. Rangel-Frausto MS, Pittet D, Costigan M, Hwang T, Davis CS, Wenzel RP (1995) The natural history of the systemic inflammatory response syndrome (SIRS). JAMA 273: 117–123
32. Schaer GL, Mitchell PF, Chernow B, Ahmed S, Parrillo JE (1990) Renal hemodynamics and prostaglandin E2 excretion in a nonhuman primate model of septic shock. Crit Care Med 18: 52–59
33. Schaller MD, Waeber D, Nussberger J, Brunner HR (1985) Angiotensin II, vasopressin and sympathetic activity in conscious rats with endotoxemia. Am J Physiol 249: H1086–H1092
34. Schaub RG, Ochoa R, Simmons CA, Lincoln KL (1987) Renal microthrombosis following endotoxin infusion may be mediated by lipoxygenase products. Circ Shock 21: 261–270

35. Voerman HJ, Stehouwer CDA, van Kamp GJ, Strack van Schijndel RJM, Groeneveld ABJ, Thijs LG (1992) Plasma endothelin levels are increased during septic shock. Crit Care Med 20:1097–1101
36. Walker JF, Cumming AD, Lindsay RM, Solez K, Linton AL (1986) The renal response produced by nonhypotensive sepsis in a large animal model. Am J Kid Dis 8:88–97
37. Willam C, Schindler R, Frei U, Eckardt KU (1999) Increases in oxygen tension stimulate the expression of ICAM-1 and VCAM-1 on human endothelial cells. Am J Physiol 276:H2044–2052
38. Zager RA, Altschuld R (1986) Body temperature: an important determinant of severity of ischemic renal injury. Am J Physiol 251:F87–F93
39. Zager RA, Prior RB (1986) Gentamycin and gram-negative bacteremia. J Clin Invest 78:196–204

CHAPTER 11

Cardiac Complications of Septicemia

A. Mebazaa

Septic shock is a highly lethal syndrome characterized by a multiple organ dysfunction [1, 2]. The latter includes myocardial dysfunction that appears in the very early phase of sepsis and is characterized by decreased indices of myocardial contraction, a tendency to increase end-diastolic volumes and affecting both the right and left ventricles. Sepsis-induced myocardial dysfunction is paradoxically associated with a high cardiac output. Interrestingly, septic cardiomyopathy starts to improve 3–5 days after the treatment of the infection and is totally resolved a few days later.

Alteration in Systolic Function

Because of the increased cardiac output and the marked alterations in hemodynamic load and heart rate, myocardial dysfunction was only recently recognized in human septic shock. In 1984, an early alteration in myocardial contraction was demonstrated by the use of radionuclide cineangiography and pulmonary artery catheter in septic patients [3, 4]. It was described as a "paradoxical" decrease in left ventricular ejection fraction while left ventricular afterload was reduced [3–5]. Ognibene et al. studied the preload-stoke volume index (SWI = stoke volume × mean arterial blood pressure/body surface area) relation that is a better estimate of the Frank-Starling relation and left ventricular function [6]. These authors showed a down- and rightward shift of this relation suggesting a depressed left ventricular function in septic patients. In addition, left ventricular systolic elastance that truly reflects systolic function was consistently reduced in several animal models of sepsis [7, 8]. A similar decrease in right ventricular function was also observed [3].

Alteration in Diastolic Function

A decreased ventricular compliance was suggested in septic patients by the measurements of transmitral and pulmonary venous flows using Doppler technique [9]. More globally, several authors found a biventricular dilation in septic humans and animals. These data are, however, controversial [3, 10, 11]. Ventricular dilation in septic patients was only seen when fluid challenge exceeded 15 l/day. This is unusual in European ICUsand may explain why several authors, mostly Europeans, could not confirm the existence of ventricular dilation in septic patients [12].

Myocardial Depressant Factors

The first suggested mechanism of sepsis-induced myocardial depression appeared to be a direct negative inotropic effects of various circulating factors produced by various cells, including bacteria, white blood cells, and endothelial cells. In 1970, it was shown that the plasma of septic animals alters the contractility of normal heart tissu in vitro [13]. A similar effect was observed with serum of septic patients incubated with cat cardiac myocytes [14]. The potential circulating depressant factor appears to have a molecular weight of < 2000 daltons.

Bacterial endotoxins that are lipopolysaccharide (LPS) contained in the cell membrane of Gram negative bacteria and released during infection may mimic septic shock in humans [15]. LPS administration in human volunteers induces a decrease in left ventricular ejection fraction that develops over 3–5 h. The time course of the onset of cardiovascular effects suggests that endotoxin does not have a direct effect by itself but, instead, that cardiovascular alterations could be related to the transient rise in the plasma levels of cytokines.

Cytokines play a key role in initiating the effective anti-infectious process while anti-inflammatory cytokines are involved in the control of the inflammatory process amplitude [16]. In addition to their immunologic effects, cytokines have some harmful effects that can lead to multiple organ dysfunction. Cytokines such as tumor necrosis factor α (TNF-α, interleukin 1β, 2 and 6, and interferon γ are known to mimic sepsis-induced hemodynamic alterations [2]. These cytokines alter myocardial function either directly or indirectly via an increased myocardial nitric oxide (NO) production [1]. Thus, TNFα was shown to induce a negative inotropic effects that was reversed by an NOS blocking agent. However, the role of NO on myocardial effect of TNFα appears to be controversial.

Intrinsic Alteration of Myocardial Properties

Since sepsis-induced myocardial dysfunction persists ex vivo, several authors suggested that alteration in cardiac intrinsic properties is a key mechanism [1]. Myocardial dysfunction can be seen in isolated heart, papillary muscle or isolated cardiomycytes from septic animals.

Several mechanisms have been suggested, including an alteration in cardiac myofilament properties and the adenylyl cyclase pathway. Several authors demonstrated that the decrease in systolic properties might be related to a decrease in cardiac myofilament response to calcium [2, 17]. In isolated rat cardiac myocytes, we showed that sepsis induces a decrease in cell shortening with no changes in intracellular calcium concentrations. Tavernier et al. showed that myofilament calcium sensitivity was decreased in skinned fibers taken from LPS-treated rabbits [17]. Stimulation of protein kinase C by isoproterenol pretreatment confirms that, during endotoxemia, protein phosphorylation decreases myofibrillar calcium sensitivity. This may contribute to sepsis-induced myocardial dysfunction.

In parallel, the adenylyl cyclase pathway is altered [18]. Several studies showed that exposure of isolated cardiac myocytes to endotoxin, cytokines, or conditioned medium from endotoxin-stimulated macrophages causes a marked reduction in cardiac myocyte contractile responsiveness to β-agonist. In addition, the total number of α and β adrenergic receptors undergoes a biphasic change following caecal ligation in vivo [19, 20]. Receptors density increases in the early phase of sepsis while it is reduced in the late phase of sepsis. Sensitization of β-receptors is also observed in the early phase of sepsis. This sensitization disappears in the late phase of sepsis.

Several pieces of evidence suggest that an overproduction of NO in cardiac myocytes and microvascular, coronary, and endocardial endothelial cells may directly contribute to the alteration of myocardial function during sepsis [21]. This hypothesis was based on functional data. Brady et al. showed that the reduced fractional shortening measured in isolated cardiac myocytes from endotoxemic guinea pig was reversed by L-NAME [22]. These data are somewhat controversial. Recent preliminary observations from our group in a rabbit model of endotoxemia suggest that myocardial dysfunction is not related to an overproduction of NO. Decking et al also reported that, in ex vivo endotoxin-treated guinea pig isolated hearts, the alteration in contractile properties is not related to NO [23]. Neither the treatment with L-NMMA nor that with L-NAME, two inhibitors of NO synthesis, reversed myocardial depression, despite an increase in coronary perfusion pressure. Analogous findings were obtained by other groups (reviewed in [1]). In addition, administration of NOS inhibitors in septic patients induced an aggravation of cardiovascular dysfunction [2]. Accordingly, NOS inhibitors are of no use in septic patients.

In summary, septic cardiomyopathy occurs very early in the time course of sepsis. Its mechanism is mainly related to alteration in intrinsic properties of cardiac muscle including cardiac myofilament properties and β-adrenergic pathway. A role for a myocardial overproduction of NO remains controversial.

References

1. Corda SA, Mebazaa B, Tavernier M, Ben Ayed M, Payen D (1998) Paracrine regulation of cardiac myocytes in normal and septic heart. J Crit Care 13:39–47
2. Grocott-Mason R, Shah A (1998) Cardiac dysfunction in sepsis: new theories and clinical implications. Int Care Med 24:286–295
3. Kimchi A, Ellrodt A, Berman D, Riedinger M, Swan H, Murata G (1984) Right venricular performance in septic shock: a combined radionuclide and hemodynamic study. J Am Coll Cardiol 1984:945–951
4. Parker, M, Shelhamer J, B. SL. (1984) Profound but reversible myocardial depression in patients with septic shock. Ann Int Med 100:483–490
5. Ozier, Y, Gueret P, Jardin F, Farcot J, Bourdarias J, Margairaz A (1984) Two-dimensional echocardiographic demonstration of acute myocardial depression in septic shock. Crit Care Med 12:596–599
6. Ognibene F, Parker M, Natanson C, Shelhamer J, Parillo J (1988) Depressed left ventricular performance. Response to volume infusion in patients with sepsis and septic shock. Chest 93:903–910
7. Hung J, Lew W (1993) Temporal sequence of endotoxin -induced systolic and diastolic myocardial depression in rabbits. Am J Physiol 265:H810-H819
8. Hung J, Lew W (1993) Cellular mechanisms of endotoxin-induced myocardial depression in rabbits. Circ Res 73:125–134
9. Poelaert J, Declerck C, Vogelaers D, Colardyn F, Visser C (1997) Left ventricular systolic and diastolic function in septic shock. Int Care Med 23:553–560
10. Natanson C, Fink M, Ballantyne H, Mac Vittie T, Conklin J, Parillo J (1986) Gram-negative bacteremia produces both severe systolic and diastolic cardiac dysfunction in a canine model that simulates human septic shock. J Clin Invest 78:259–270
11. Parker M, Natanson C, Suffredini R, Danner R, Cunnion R, Ognibene F, Parrillo J (1990) Septic shock in humans: advances in the understanding of pathogenesis, cardiovascular dysfunction and therapy. Ann Intern Med 113:227–242
12. Jardin F, Brun-Ney D, Auvert B, Beauchet A, Bourdarias J (1990) Sepsis-related cardiogenic shock. Crit Care Med 18:1055–1060
13. Lefer A (1970) Role of a myocardial depressant factor in the pathogenesis of circulatory shock. Fed Proc 29:1836–1847
14. Parrillo J, Burch C, Shelhamer J, Parker M, Natanson C, Schuette W (1985) A circulating myocardial depressant substance in humans with septic shock. J Clin Invest 76:1539–1553

15. Suffredini A, Fromm R, Parker M, Brenner M, Kovacs J, Wesley R, Parrillo J (1989) The cardiovascular response of normal humans to the administration of endotoxin. N Engl J Med 321:280–287
16. Bone R, Grodzin C, Balk R (1997) Sepsis: a new hypothesis for pathogenesis of disease process. Chest 112:235–243
17. Tavernier B, Garrigue D, Boulle C, Vallet B, Adnet P (1998) Myofilament calcium sensitivity is decreased in skinned cardiac fibres of endotoxin-treated rabbits. Cardiovasc Res 38:472–479
18. Tavernier B, Abi-Gerges N, Mebazaa A (1999) Alteration of the beta-adrenergic pathway in the septic heart. In: Yearbook of Intensive Care and Emergency Medicine 1999. Edited by J-L Vincent. Springer, Berlin Heidelberg New York, pp 504–518
19. Tang C, Liu M (1996) Initial externalization followed by internalization of β-adrenergic receptors in rat heart during sepsis. Am J Physiol 270:R254-R263
20. Wu L, Tang C, Liu M (1997) Hyper- and hypocardiodynamic states are associated with externalization and internalization, respectively, of α-adrenergic receptors in rat heart during sepsis. Shock 7:318–322
21. Kelly R, Balligand J, Smith T (1996) Nitric oxide and cardiac function. Circ Res 79: 363–380
22. Brady A, Poole-Wilson P, Harding S, Warren J (1992) Nitric oxide production within cardiac myocytes reduces their contractility in endotoxemia. Am J Physiol 263:H1963-H1966
23. Decking U, Flesche C, Godecke A, Schrader J (1995) Endotoxin-induced contractile dysfunction in guinea pig hearts is not mediated by nitric oxide. Am J Physiol 268:H2460-H2465

Sachverzeichnis

Computer to Film: Saladruck, Berlin
Binding: Buchbinderei Lüderitz & Bauer, Berlin